MEDICAL BOARDS STEP 3
made ridiculously simple

Andreas Carl, M.D., Ph.D.
Adjunct Assistant Professor
University Nevada School of Medicine
Department of Physiology and Cell Biology
Reno, NV 89557-0046

MedMaster, Inc., Miami

ISBN # 0-940780-54-2

Made in the United States of America

Published by
MedMaster, Inc.
P.O. Box 640028
Miami, FL 33164

for Dr. Victor Ruiz-Velasco

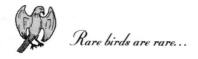 *Rare birds are rare...*

PREFACE TO THE 2nd EDITION

The USMLE Step 3 has changed significantly since I wrote the 1st edition of this book and has become more difficult than it used to be. You cannot rely on simple "high-yield-facts" anymore and a thorough understanding of patient management and prioritization is most important. Computer-based case simulations now account for about 25% of your score. I have completely rewritten this book for the new USMLE Step 3 format and the old chapter 2 (Preventive Medicine and Epidemiology) has been replaced with **Patient Management.** Most information is presented in a simple step-by-step approach.

I wish to thank the many students whose input has allowed me to keep this book current and relevant for the USMLE exam.

Please visit my web-site to share your experiences with other students:

www.usmle.net

If you are about to take the exam or just took it, you can contact me via e-mail:

andreas@usmle.net

USMLE STEP 3 FORMAT

Compared to the Step 2 exam, questions tend to be more complex, more information is presented and it will take longer to read through the cases. I always recommend to read the last sentence of each case presentation, to get an idea what the question is about. This way you can read more selectively and extract the useful information.

All questions are single best choice and arranged in settings:

- Satellite Health Center
- Office
- Hospital
- Emergency Department.

While this format is intended to make the exam more "realistic" you will find that it has surprisingly little effect on your actual test taking. You still will have to answer each question based on solely the information presented in each case.

Many questions on the USMLE Step 3 exam end with a phrase like "the most appropriate next step would be to...", "the most appropriate intervention would be..." and similar phrases. My *Medical Boards Step 3 Made Ridiculously Simple* gives you exact information in a step-by-step fashion to help you answer this type of questions.

WHICH BOOK SHOULD I USE?

You should use the same materials you already used for your Step 2 preparation since you are familiar with these and it makes for the most efficient review. If you have used my *Medical Boards Step 2 Made Ridiculously Simple* book - great! I strongly recommend you take a day or two and go over the charts presented there. About 10% of the questions on the Step 3 exam are Basic Science and it is important to review the Pharmacology and Pathology Chapters from my Step 1 book. For additional updated information about popular study aids, please visit my web-site.

WHAT IS THE DIFFERENCE BETWEEN THIS *STEP 3* AND MY *STEP 2* BOOK?

Medical Boards Step 3 Made Ridiculously Simple is the perfect companion to my *Medical Boards Step 2 Made Ridiculously Simple* book. While the Step 2 book presents material in a "disease-oriented approach" centered around organ systems, the Step 3 book presents material in a more "patient-oriented approach".

The two books are designed to go "hand-in-hand" and complement each other. The Step 2 book will give you a solid foundation to pass the Step 2 exam and also would serve you well for the Step 3. My *Medical Boards Step 3 Made Ridiculously Simple* extends the material in areas which are emphasized on the USMLE Step 3 exam, namely diagnostic approaches and patient management. You can use *Medical Boards Step 3 Made Ridiculously Simple* together with my Step 2 book or to supplement other review books you like to use.

All areas of Medicine are covered in both books, however the emphasis is different:

STEP 2 book	**STEP 3 book**
• Diseases and Organ Systems	• Diagnosis, Step-by-Step • Patient Management

HOW TO USE THIS BOOK?

Chapter 1 presents a step-by-step approach to medical diagnosis, beginning with a symptom or sign followed by diagnostic tests arranged systematically from top to bottom in flow-charts. The diagnostic tests presented at the top of each charts are the least invasive and typically give the highest yield.

The tests at the bottom of each chart are the most invasive with the lowest yield. You should pay careful attention to the order of these tests. It is assumed that you work your way from top to bottom, proceeding to the next test, if the results from the previous one were negative.

Chapter 2 presents patient management in a similar Step-by-Step fashion. You need to know about risk factors and prevention of disease and simple treatment algorithms. Please keep in mind that *Medical Boards Step 3 Made Ridiculously Simple* is not a textbook. Rather, facts are presented in a logical and easily accessible format in order to help you review the key facts just prior to the exam.

Both chapters are arranged in alphabetical fashion for easy reference. For Students and Residents who have the time and wish to prepare themselves in a more systematic way, a **Table of Contents by Organ Systems** is provided. It is hoped that this book will not only be useful for your exam preparation but also as a quick refresher during your clinical years. How you score on the USMLE Step 3 exam not only depends on how hard you study, but also on what you study. Obviously, if you study what they ask, you will achieve a very high score. Care has been taken not to overload this book with "rare birds"...

> ➤ Use it during your clinical work to organize your thoughts
> ➤ Use it as a refresher course
> ➤ Use it as a last minute review

IMPORTANT DISCLAIMER:

The diagnostic and therapeutic algorithms in this book are meant as examples only and not for treatment of actual patients. Real-world medicine is more complicated than what can be presented in a book like this. The purpose of these diagnostic and therapeutic algorithms is to remind you of common approaches to typical medical problems you may encounter on the USMLE Step 3 exam. When treating a patient, you will often deviate from any such schematics, depending on the individual case. Always treat the patient, not the symptoms!

I wish to thank Steve Goldberg for the cartoons. I hope that this text will help your preparation for the USMLE Step 3 and would appreciate any comments about the selection and presentation of this material you might have. Good luck!

www.usmle.net
- ➤ latest trends on the USMLE
- ➤ bulletin board
- ➤ book recommendations

REFERENCES

1. Cecil Textbook of Medicine, W.B. Saunders Co.
2. Current Medical Diagnosis&Treatment, Appleton&Lange
3. Current Emergency Diagnosis&Treatment, Appleton&Lange
4. Current Obstetric&Gynecologic Diagnosis&Treatment, Appleton&Lange
5. Current Pediatric Diagnosis&Treatment, Appleton&Lange
6. Decision Making in Medicine, Mosby
7. Dermatology in General Medicine, McGraw-Hill
8. Harrison's Principles of Internal Medicine, McGraw-Hill
9. Heart Disease - A Textbook of Cardiovascular Medicine, W.B. Saunders Co.
10. Internal Medicine, Ed. J.H. Stein, Mosby
11. Mayo Internal Medicine Board Review, Mayo Foundation
12. Obstetrics and Gynecology, J.B. Lippincott Co.
13. Principles and Practice of Infectious Diseases, Churchill Livingstone
14. Principles of Neurology, McGraw-Hill
15. Rudolph's Pediatrics, Appleton&Lange
16. Synopsis of Psychiatry, Williams&Wilkins
17. Williams Hematology, McGraw-Hill

CONTENTS

TABLE OF CONTENTS BY ORGAN SYSTEMS

GENERAL SYMPTOMS AND SIGNS

ELECTROLYTE IMBALANCES

CARDIOVASCULAR DISEASES

RESPIRATORY DISEASES

GASTROINTESTINAL DISEASES

ENDOCRINE DISEASES

MUSCULOSKELETAL DISEASES

DISEASES OF THE EYE AND SKIN

OBSTETRICS & GYNECOLOGY

PEDIATRIC DISEASES

INFECTIOUS DISEASES

MALIGNANCIES

NEUROLOGICAL DISEASES

PSYCHIATRIC DISEASES

DIAGNOSIS

STEP by STEP

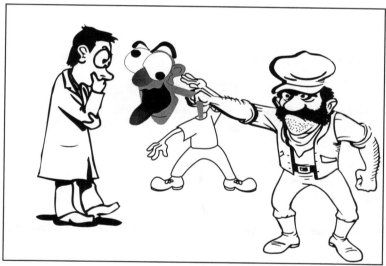

"Hmm.... could be hyperthyroidism"

1.1.) <u>ACUTE ABDOMEN</u>

1. If unstable:
get surgical consultation → laparotomy
- perforation
- hemorrhage
- bowel obstruction
- bowel infarction

2. If stable:
you must rule out:
- myocardial infarction
- lower lobe pneumonia
- pancreatitis
- pyelonephritis

3. If none of the above, you should consider:
- hepatitis
- peritonitis
- diabetic ketoacidosis
- Addisonian crisis
- acute intermittent porphyria

1.2.) <u>ABDOMINAL PAIN - UPPER</u>

1. Get ECG and chest X-ray
- myocardial infarction
- pericarditis
- pleuritis
- lower lobe pneumonia

2. Get upright abdominal film
- free air → perforation
- opacities → gall stones
- dilated bowel → obstruction or infarction

3. Get chemistry
- amylase, lipase → acute pancreatitis
- transaminases → viral or hepatocellular disease

4. Consider ultrasound
- acute cholecystitis
- hepatic abscess
- subphrenic abscess

5. Consider upper GI endoscopy / ERCP
- gastroesophageal reflux disease
- peptic ulcer
- biliary disease

1.3.) ABDOMINAL PAIN - PERIUMBILICAL

1. Get abdominal flat plate or ultrasound
if evidence of intestinal obstruction, search for:
- strangulation
- adhesions
- tumors
- regional enteritis

otherwise consider:
- bowel infarction
- aortic aneurysm

2. Get barium contrast enema
- appendicitis
- diverticulitis

3. If none of the above, you should consider:
- Meckel's diverticulitis
- acute intermittent porphyria
- lead intoxication

Irritable bowel syndrome is the most common cause of chronic abdominal pain:
- at least during 12 weeks for past 12 months
- change in school frequency or appearance
- relieved after defecation

1.4.) <u>ABDOMINAL PAIN - LOWER</u>

1. **Perform pelvic and rectal exam**
   - ovarian cysts or tumors
   - salpingitis
   - ectopic pregnancy
   - rectal carcinoma

2. **Consider barium contrast enema**
   - appendicitis, diverticulitis
   - inflammatory bowel disease

3. **Consider IVP**
   - ureteral stone or tumor

4. **Consider bladder catheterization**
   - if distended → obstruction

5. **Consider sigmoidoscopy**
   - sigmoid carcinoma
   - inflammatory bowel disease
   - diverticulitis

If none of the above:
   - Irritable bowel syndrome

In females of reproductive age with acute abdominal pain get a pregnancy test. If positive, verify intrauterine location with ultrasound to exclude ectopic pregnancy.

1.5.) <u>ACIDOSIS</u>
(pH < 7.35)

respiratory acidosis (PCO_2 >40 mmHg, HCO_3 >24 mM/L)	• hypoventilation • decreased gas exchange • airway obstruction

metabolic acidosis
(PCO_2 <40 mmHg, HCO_3 <24 mM/L)
anion gap > 12 mM/L
	drug history
	• salicylate intoxication
	• methanol ingestion
	• ethylene glycol
	
	ketones present
	• glucose > 200 mg/dL
	   → diabetic ketoacidosis
	• glucose < 200 mg/dL
	   → starvation
	
	ketones absent
	• renal failure
	• lactic acidosis

metabolic acidosis
  (PCO_2 <40 mmHg, HCO_3 <24 mM/L)
  anion gap < 12 mM/L
 	
= "hyperchloremic metabolic acidosis"
	urine pH > 5.5
	renal loss of bicarbonate
	• carbonic anhydrase inhibitors
	• renal tubular acidosis
	• hypoaldosteronism
	
	urine pH < 5.5
	GI loss of bicarbonate
	• diarrhea
	• ileostomy

1.6.) <u>AGITATION</u>

outburst of rage and violence	could be another episode in a lifelong sequence of sociopathic behavior…
rage and violence a/w seizure activity	• temporal lobe seizures • amygdala seizures [1]
extreme freight, agitation	**delirium** • clouded consciousness • psychomotor overactivity • hallucinations **schizophrenia** • delusions **anxiety disorder** • acute panic attack
depression, anxiety, bizarre ideation,	**developing over months or years:** • schizophrenia • manic-depressive disorder

[1] *may be triggered by small amounts of alcohol*

1.7.) AIDS

(acquired immunodeficiency syndrome)

Definition (CDC revised 1993)

HIV positive on ELISA and confirmed by Western blot

plus • CD4 < 200 cells/mm³
       • or CD4 < 14%
       • or opportunistic disease

Acute retroviral syndrome : - fever
                          - lymphadenopathy
                          - pharyngitis
                          - rash
                          - myalgia
                          - thrombocytopenia
                          - leukopenia

CD4 count : - check every 6 months if CD4 > 300
                   - check every 3 months if CD4 < 300
                   - start PCP prophylaxis if CD4 < 200

ELISA	• detects antibodies against HIV • sensitivity and specificity are >99% • positive result needs to be confirmed by Western blot
p24 antigen	• for diagnosis of acute infection • not very sensitive
PCR	• detects smallest amount of viral material

1.8.) ALKALINE PHOSPHATASE
(>105 U/L)

high 5' nucleotidase high γGT	• biliary disease • liver disease ○ metastases ○ hepatocellular carcinoma
high serum calcium low serum phosphate	• osteomalacia
X-ray skull	• Paget's disease
technetium bone scan	• bone tumors • metastatic disease
other	• pregnancy

γGT is elevated in 97% of patients with liver metastases.

γGT is the most sensitive marker of liver damage due to alcohol.

Alkaline phosphatase isoenzymes (electrophoresis) are more difficult and expensive than the indirect methods to distinguish liver disease from bone disease.

1.9.) <u>ALKALOSIS</u>
(pH > 7.45)

respiratory alkalosis (PCO_2 <35 mmHg, HCO_3 <25 mM/L)	**hypoxia** • altitude sickness **central stimulation** • anxiety → hyperventilation • salicylate intoxication • encephalitis
metabolic alkalosis (PCO_2 >40 mmHg, HCO_3 >28 mM/L) **urine Cl < 10 mM/L**	**GI loss of acid** • vomiting • nasogastric suction
metabolic alkalosis (PCO_2 >40 mmHg, HCO_3 >28 mM/L) **urine Cl > 15 mM/L**	**high blood pressure:** • hyperaldosteronism • Cushing's syndrome • renal artery stenosis **normal blood pressure:** • Bartter's syndrome • severe K^+ deficit • diuretics

 Hypovolemia prevents renal bicarbonate formation.

<u>Salicylate intoxication:</u>
Early: metabolic acidosis + respiratory alkalosis
Late: metabolic acidosis + respiratory acidosis

1.10.) ALOPECIA

1. If scarring is present → do biopsy first!

Infections:
- syphilis

systemic diseases:
- discoid lupus
- scleroderma/morphea
- amyloidosis
- sarcoidosis
- (many more)

neoplasms:
- skin cancer
- metastatic cancer
- lymphoma

2. If no scarring → screen for these:

- **thyroid function tests:** hypothyroidism, hyperthyroidism
- **VDRL:** syphilis
- **ferritin < 10 ng/mL:** iron deficiency
- **ANA:** SLE

3. also consider:
- malnutrition
- trichotillomania
- drugs

1.11.) ALTERED MENTAL STATE

1. Is there a history of trauma? → get CT or MRI
CT scan abnormal:
- subdural hematoma
- intracranial bleed

CT scan normal:
- concussion

2. Initial workup:
- body temperature → hypo/hyperthermia, sepsis
- EKG → arrhythmias
- ABG → hypoxia, hypercapnia, CO
- electrolytes → hypo-/hypernatremia

- metabolites → hyperglycemia
  hypoglycemia
  uremia
  liver failure
  thyroid storm

3. If negative, consider:
- toxic screen → drugs, toxins
- EEG → petit mal seizure, postictal state
- lumbar puncture → meningitis, encephalitis
  subarachnoid bleed
- CT or MRI → intracranial bleed

- Get psychiatric evaluation !

1.12.) <u>SECONDARY AMENORRHEA</u>
<u>NORMAL PROLACTIN</u>

1. Exclude Pregnancy !!!

2. Check TSH levels → hypothyroidism

3. Perform Progesterone Challenge

withdrawal bleeding → **anovulation**
        polycystic ovarian disease
        adrenal tumor
        ovarian tumor

4. Perform Estrogen-Progesterone Challenge

withdrawal bleeding →   **high LH / FSH**
        ovarian failure

        normal or low LH / FSH
        get head CT or MRI (see 1.13.):
        if normal: hypothalamic amenorrhea

no withdrawal bleeding →   **outflow tract problem**
        Asherman's syndrome
        active endometritis

*Any women with primary ovarian failure or ovarian failure
before age 35 ("premature menopause") should be karyotyped.*

13

1.13.) <u>SECONDARY AMENORRHEA</u>
<u>PROLACTIN > 20 ng/mL</u>

1. Exclude Pregnancy !!!

2. Get drug history
- phenothiazines
- monoamine inhibitors
- tricyclic antidepressants

3. Get head CT or MRI → pituitary lesions
- adenoma
- craniopharyngioma
- Sheehan's syndrome
- empty sella syndrome

4. If CT or MRI normal → hypothalamic amenorrhea
- exercise
- stress
- anorexia nervosa

Hypothalamic amenorrhea *is a diagnosis of exclusion. It is the most common cause of secondary amenorrhea in non-pregnant women. Prolactin levels may be normal or elevated.*

1.14.) <u>AMNESIA</u>

A) <u>SUDDEN ONSET</u>:

complete recovery	<ul><li>post-concussion</li><li>TIA to hippocampal areas [1]</li><li>temporal lobe seizures</li></ul>
incomplete recovery	<ul><li>hippocampal infarction</li><li>thalamic infarction</li><li>subarachnoid hemorrhage</li><li>prolonged hypoxia</li></ul>

B) <u>SLOW ONSET</u>:

incomplete recovery	<ul><li>Wernicke-Korsakoff syndrome [2]</li><li>encephalitis</li></ul>
no recovery	<ul><li>Alzheimer's disease</li><li>diencephalic tumors</li></ul>

[1] *patient may wonder "where am I, what's happening?"*

[2] *memory gaps are filled in with fantastic stories (confabulation)*

1.15.) <u>MICROCYTIC ANEMIA</u>
(MCV < 82 fL)

TIBC - high ferritin - low iron - low	**iron deficiency** • infants: decreased dietary intake • elderly: occult bleed (especially GI) • other: malabsorption
TIBC - low **ferritin** **- high** iron - low	• anemia of chronic disease [1]
TIBC - normal **ferritin** **- high** **iron** **- high**	**blocked heme synthesis** • lead poisoning • sideroblastic anemia
electrophoresis	• sickle cell anemia • thalassemia

[1] *can be microcytic or normocytic*

16

1.16.) NORMOCYTIC ANEMIA
(MCV 82-98 fL)

reticulocytes > 1.5%	• blood loss • hemolytic anemia
MCHC > 36 g/dL	• hereditary spherocytosis
bone marrow biopsy	**hypoplasia** • aplastic anemia **myelophthisis** [1] • myeloma • lymphoma • leukemia • granulomatous disease • lipid storage disease **erythroid hyperplasia** • early iron deficiency
other	• chronic liver disease • chronic renal disease

[1] *myelophthisis = infiltration and replacement of bone marrow*

1.17.) <u>MACROCYTIC ANEMIA</u>
(MCV > 98 fL)

B12 < 160 pg/mL	**absolute B12 deficiency** • pernicious anemia • malabsorption • ileal resection
folate < 2 ng/mL	**absolute folate deficiency** • ethanol • dietary
bone marrow biopsy	**normoblastic** • hemolysis • chronic liver disease **megaloblastic** • relative B12 deficiency • relative folate deficiency **myelodysplasia** • refractory anemia etc. • CMML

1.18.) HEMOLYTIC ANEMIA

direct Coombs' test positive	indirect Coombs' test positive: • hemolytic disease of newborn • transfusion reaction indirect Coombs' test negative: • warm antibodies • cold antibodies
membrane abnormalities	• spherocytosis • elliptocytosis
metabolic abnormalities	• glucose-6-PD deficiency
hemoglobin abnormalities	• sickle cell anemia • thalassemia
mechanical trauma	• march hemoglobinuria • artificial heart valves • DIC
other	• burns • chemicals • hypersplenism

WARM ANTIBODIES	COLD ANTIBODIES
• drugs • infections • collagen vascular diseases • multiple myeloma • lymphoma	• mononucleosis • mycoplasma infection • multiple myeloma • lymphoma • paroxysmal cold hemoglobinuria

1.19.) APLASTIC ANEMIA

drugs: dose related (predictable)	➤ chloramphenicol • benzene • chemotherapy
drugs: not dose related (unpredictable)	➤ chloramphenicol ➤ phenylbutazone ➤ sulfa drugs ➤ amantadine ➤ ACE inhibitors
hereditary	• Fanconi's anemia
other	• infections • radiation

1.20.) ANXIETY

drugs	➢ drug abuse ➢ medications
medical conditions	• cardiac arrhythmias • hyperthyroidism • pheochromocytoma
objects, situations	• specific phobia • social phobia • separation anxiety
severe traumatic event	**duration < 1 month:** • acute stress disorder **duration > 1 month:** • post-traumatic stress disorder
obsessions	• obsessive-compulsive disorder
recurrent panic attacks + constant worry about attacks + behavioral changes to avoid these attacks	• agoraphobia

1.21.) ARTHRALGIA

A) INVOLVING SEVERAL JOINTS:

1. If spine is not involved, you should consider:
- rheumatoid arthritis
- psoriatic arthritis
- SLE

2. If spine is involved, you should consider:
- ankylosing spondylitis
- Reiter's syndrome

B) INVOLVING ONE JOINT:

Perform arthrocentesis:

1. If non-inflammatory
- bloody effusion → trauma or coagulopathy
- non-bloody effusion → osteoarthritis

2. If inflammatory (synovial WBC usually > 50,000)
- look for crystals:
  positive birefringence → pseudogout
  negative birefringence → gout

3. Get Gram stain or culture of synovial fluid
- infectious arthritis
  (common causes: syphilis or Lyme disease)

1.22.) ASCITES

A) <u>TRANSUDATE</u> (protein < 2.5 g/dL):

1. Check for signs of portal hypertension
- liver cirrhosis
- congestive heart failure
- IVC obstruction

▼

2. Check albumin levels
- nephrotic syndrome
- malnutrition

▼

3. Evidence of abdominal neoplasms? (Meig's syndrome)
- ovarian fibroma
- ovarian cystadenoma
- struma ovarii

B) <u>EXUDATE</u> (protein > 2.5 g/dL):

1. Check PMN count - if >250:
- peritonitis
  (bacterial, tuberculosis, or fungal)

▼

2. Check cytology
- hepatoma, mesothelioma
- ovarian carcinoma
- metastatic carcinoma

▼

3. Check amylase levels
- pancreatitis

1.23.) <u>BLEEDING</u>

platelets < 100,000	• thrombocytopenia
PT prolonged	• Factor VII deficiency • vitamin K deficiency • liver disease
PTT prolonged	• Von Willebrand's disease • Factor VIII (hemophilia A) • Factor IX (hemophilia B) o circulating anticoagulants
both PT and PTT prolonged	➤ heparin • vitamin K deficiency • liver failure • DIC o dysfibrinogenemia o circulating anticoagulants
bleeding time prolonged > 10 min	• platelet dysfunction o myeloproliferative disorders o uremia

<u>Mixing Studies:</u>
(repeat PT, PTT with equal mixture of patient's and "normal" plasma)

if times correct   → factor deficiency
if times do not correct → factor inhibition

1.24.) <u>BRADYCARDIA</u>
(< 60 beats/min)

---

1. Check drug history for causes of bradycardia
- digitalis
- beta-blockers
- calcium antagonists

↓

2. Obtain an ECG

- **1st degree AV block**
  PR > 0.2 sec.
- **2nd degree AV block, Mobitz I**
  progressive prolongation of PR
- **2nd degree AV block, Mobitz II**
  irregular, unexpected AV block
- **3rd degree AV block 1**
  complete block

↓

3. Consider Holter monitoring
- sick sinus syndrome

↓

4. His bundle ECG to determine the need for pacemaker is recommended for patients with:
- symptomatic bundle branch block
- 2:1 AV conduction block
- asymptomatic 3rd degree AV block

Trained athletes may have <50 beats/min due to increased vagal tone.

1.25.) BREAST NODULE

1. If you have a low index of suspicion, observe for:
- physiologic nodularity
- cyclic tenderness

2. If a cyst is likely:
- aspiration of fluid will be diagnostic

3. If there is a palpable lump:
→ perform fine needle aspiration (FNA)
(sensitive and specific)

4. An open breast biopsy is indicated if:
- a suspicious mass persists through cycle and an equivocal FNA.

- residual component left after attempted cyst aspiration.

- suspicious mass plus spontaneous serosanguineous discharge.

- suspicious mammogram without prominent palpable mass.

Recommend monthly breast self-examination for all women above 20 years of age.

1.26.) CARDIAC MURMURS - I

mitral stenosis	diastolic opening snap diastolic rumble loud S1 no S3 or S4 • dyspnea, orthopnea • atrial fibrillation
mitral regurgitation	holosystolic murmur may radiate to axilla widely split S2 (early A2) • pulmonary congestion
mitral valve prolapse	midsystolic click followed by murmur • palpitations • atypical chest pain
aortic stenosis	harsh systolic ejection murmur may radiate to carotids • angina • exertional syncope
aortic regurgitation	diastolic decrescendo murmur • "waterhammer pulse" DeMusset: head bobbing Traube: pistol shot sounds over arteries Quincke: pulsatile blushing of nail beds

 Follow up with - echocardiogram
- cardiac catheterization

27

1.27.) CARDIAC MURMURS - II

 Inspiration: - increases venous return
- increases right-sided murmurs

	OCM	AS	MR
Valsalva (decreases venous return)	↑	↓	↓
squatting (increases systemic vascular resistance) (increases venous return)	↓	↑	↑
amyl nitrate (decreases arterial pressure) (increases cardiac output)	↑	↑	↓

OCM: obstructive cardiomyopathy, AS: aortic stenosis, MR: mitral regurgitation
↑ : increases murmur,   ↓ : decreases murmur

physiologic split	P closes after A (inspiratory split)
wide split	P closes after A (inspiratory >> expiratory) • pulmonary stenosis • mitral regurgitation • RBBB
paradoxical split	A closes after P (expiratory split) • aortic stenosis • tricuspid regurgitation • LBBB
fixed split	split independent of respiration • ASD, VSD

1.28.) CARDIOMEGALY

echocardiogram: hypertrophy	**asymmetrical** • hypertrophic cardiomyopathy **symmetrical** • hypertension • coarctation of aorta • high-output state
echocardiogram: dilation	**left ventricle** • decompensation **aortic stenosis** • left ventricle and aorta • aortic regurgitation **left ventricle and left atrium** • mitral regurgitation **left atrium and pulmonary artery** • mitral stenosis **right ventricle, "pruning" of pulmonary vessels** • cor pulmonale • primary pulmonary hypertension **generalized enlargement** • alcohol abuse • post viral
echocardiogram: pericardial	• pericardial effusion • infiltrative disease
echocardiogram: normal	• kyphoscoliosis • pregnancy • mediastinal mass

1.29.) CHEST PAIN

1. Check ECG for signs of ischemia
- cardiac enzymes elevated → myocardial infarction
- cardiac enzymes normal → angina pectoris

2. If arterial blood gases show hypoxemia:
get ventilation-perfusion scan:
- pulmonary embolus

get echocardiogram:
- aortic stenosis
- mitral valve prolapse
- cardiomyopathy
- pericarditis

3. Get a chest X-ray
- pneumothorax
- pneumonia
- aortic aneurysm

4. Other tests to perform if chest pain persists:

Treadmill, cardiac catheter, Holter monitor:
- coronary artery disease
- arrhythmia

Evaluate gastrointestinal tract:
- ulcer disease
- esophageal disease
- gallbladder disease

Also consider:
- skeletal pain, psychogenic pain

1.30.) CONSTIPATION

1. Check drug history for causes of constipation
- anticholinergics
  (phenothiazines, antidepressants, anticonvulsants)
- narcotics
- aluminum-containing antacids
- laxative abuse (*melanosis coli*)

2. Search for electrolytes or metabolic causes
- hypokalemia
- hypothyroidism
- diabetes mellitus

3. Perform sigmoidoscopy
- anorectal fissures/strictures/abscess
- rectal carcinoma
- diverticulitis

4. Perform barium enema or colonoscopy
- strictures
- polyps or carcinoma
if dilated → biopsy
- Hirschsprung's disease
- Chagas' disease

4. If none of the above, consider:
- irritable bowel syndrome
- depression

1.31.) COUGH

1. Check for signs of infection or allergy
- bronchitis, pharyngitis
- exposure to airway irritants

2. Chest X-ray shows a solitary lesion
- malignancy
- fungal infection

3. Chest X-ray shows diffuse infiltration
sputum culture positive
- bacterial, fungal or parasitic infection

sputum culture negative
- sarcoidosis
- interstitial fibrosis
- aspiration

4. Get pulmonary function tests
obstructive diseases
- asthma
- extrinsic compression

4. Consider bronchoscopy
- endobronchial tumor
- foreign body

*Chest X-ray is indicated if cough is chronic or if acute
without signs of upper respiratory infection.*

1.32.) CYANOSIS

A) PERIPHERAL CYANOSIS:
(tongue is red)

congenital	**lower extremities** patent ductus arteriosus
localized cyanosis **(O_2 saturation normal)**	venous thrombosis Raynaud's phenomenon acrocyanosis

B) CENTRAL CYANOSIS:
(tongue is blue)

$p_aO_2 > 50$ mmHg	methemoglobin (chocolate colored blood)
$p_aO_2 < 50$ mmHg	**p_aO_2 increases with 100% O_2** lung disease heart disease
$p_aO_2 < 50$ mmHg	**p_aO_2 does not increase with 100% O_2** primary right→left shunt Eisenmenger reaction
CXR	congestive heart failure pneumonia
V/Q scan	pulmonary embolus

polycythemia	- cyanosis becomes apparent early
anemia	- cyanosis becomes apparent late

1.33.) <u>DEMENTIA</u>

1. Are focal neurological signs present?
- CNS tumors
- lacunar stroke
- multiple sclerosis

2. Are extrapyramidal signs present?
- Parkinson's
- supranuclear palsy
- Huntington's

3. Check for metabolic abnormalities
- uremia
- thyroid function tests
- hepatic encephalopathy

4. Do some serological tests
- syphilis
- AIDS

5. Perform a toxic screen
- drugs
- alcohol
- heavy metals

6. Consider lumbar puncture
- meningitis
- encephalitis

7. If none of the above, consider:
- Jacob-Creutzfeldt disease
- Alzheimer's disease
- depression

parietotemporal atrophy *- probably Alzheimer's disease*
frontotemporal atrophy *- probably Pick's disease*

1.34.) <u>DIARRHEA - ACUTE</u>

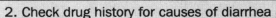

1. If no fever or systemic signs: treat symptomatically

2. Check drug history for causes of diarrhea
- laxatives
- magnesium-containing antacids
- lactulose
- antibiotics → *Cl. difficile* toxin in stool?
  (pseudomembranous colitis)

3. Check stool for ova and parasites, or culture
- *Cryptosporidium* (common in AIDS patients)
- *Giardia lamblia*
- Entamoeba histolytica
- worms

4. If stool is negative for ova and parasites:
- viral gastroenteritis

food poisoning:
- *Cl. perfringens*
- *Staph. aureus*

5. If diarrhea still persisting do sigmoidoscopy:
- rectal carcinoma
- inflammatory bowel disease

A simple test to be performed in the office is to inspect a fecal sample for WBCs/RBCs. Presence implies infection with invasive organism or inflammatory bowel disease.

1.35.) DIARRHEA - CHRONIC

1. Obtain drug history and check for ova and parasites

↓

2. Perform sigmoidoscopy or barium enema
- carcinoma
- inflammatory bowel disease
- scleroderma

↓

3. Upper GI and small bowel series or endoscopy
- Crohn's disease
- celiac sprue

↓

4. Measure fecal fat content, if > 7 g/24h:
malabsorption
- celiac sprue
- pancreatic insufficiency
- blind loop syndrome

RESULT OF A PROLONGED FAST:

DIARRHEA RESOLVES	DIARRHEA PERSISTS
D-xylose absorption test bacterial overgrowth **cholestyramine trial** bile acid malabsorption	**serum or urine hormone levels** carcinoid VIPoma

1.36.) DIZZINESS

1. Check drug history for causes of dizziness
- tranquilizers
- antihypertensives
- antidepressants

2. Consider Holter monitoring
- cardiac arrhythmia

3. Perform EEG
- seizure disorder

4. If none of the above, consider:
- posterior TIA
- hyperventilation syndrome

Vertigo   - rotating sensation
Dizziness - fainting sensation

1.37.) DYSMENORRHEA

 Colicky, labor-like pain.

1. Perform pelvic exam
- cervical stenosis
- uterine fibroids
- presence of IUD

2. Get ultrasound
- uterine abnormalities
- outflow obstructions

3. Consider hysterosalpingography or hysteroscopy
- endometrial polyps

4. Consider laparoscopy
- endometriosis
- pelvic adhesions

5. If none of the above, consider:
- "primary dysmenorrhea"
  (=absence of identifiable pelvic abnormalities)

1.38.) DYSPAREUNIA

PERFORM PHYSICAL EXAM:

vaginal opening	• residual hymen • episiotomy scar • Bartholin's gland abscess
clitoris	• irritations • infections
vagina	• infections • atrophy • decreased lubrication
uterus, tubes	• endometriosis • pelvic inflammatory disease • ectopic pregnancy
other	• psychological causes

It is not rare for a women to overcome her dyspareunia just to find her partner having become impotent...

1.39.) <u>DYSPHAGIA</u>

1. Consider esophagoscopy
- neoplasms
- esophageal rings/strictures
- Zenker's diverticulum
- achalasia

2. Consider barium swallow (video)
external compression
- mediastinal masses
- atrial enlargement

3. Consider esophageal manometry
progressive neurological disorders
- Parkinson's
- diabetic neuropathy
- multiple sclerosis
- syringomyelia

motility disorders
- scleroderma
- myasthenia gravis

---

painful swallowing: pharyngitis, stomatitis

dysphagia: sensation of impaired act of swallowing
globus: sensation that something is stuck in the throat

1.40.) DYSPNEA

CXR "pulmonary"	• pneumonia • interstitial lung disease • emphysema • pneumothorax
CXR "cardiac"	**echocardiogram** • valvular disease • myopathy
$pO_2 > 70$ mmHg	**O_2 saturation > 95%** • CO poisoning • methemoglobulinemia **hematocrit < 35%** • anemia
$pO_2 < 70$ mmHg	**V/Q scan** • pulmonary embolus **cardiac catheter** • right→left shunt • pulmonary hypertension
pulmonary function tests (PFT)	• airway obstruction • bronchospasm • restrictive disease • respiratory muscle weakness
exercise PFT	• exercise induced asthma • fixed cardiac output

1.41.) DYSPROTEINEMIA
(monoclonal gammopathy)

bone marrow abnormal (>10% plasma cells)	IgM Waldenström's macroglobulinemia [1] IgG, IgM, rarely IgA, IgD, or IgE multiple myeloma [2]
bone marrow normal (1-2% plasma cells)	IgM (secondary macroglobulinemia) chronic inflammation carcinoma lymphoma CLL urine protein electrophoresis positive primary amyloidosis [3] urine protein electrophoresis negative MGUS [4]

[1] lymphoma of medium-sized B cells
[2] malignancy of plasma cells
[3] diagnosis requires demonstration of amyloid on tissue biopsy
[4] follow monoclonal M-component with immune-electrophoresis every 6 months

---

M-component:

IgG - typical myeloma
light chain (κ or λ) - more aggressive

- may precipitate in cold (cryoglobulin) → Raynaud's
- may complex with coagulation factors → coagulopathy
- appears in urine (Bence-Jones protein) in 75% of cases

1.42.) EDEMA

A) GENERALIZED:

jugular vein pressure elevated	**echocardiogram** • congestive heart failure • pericarditis • tamponade
serum albumin < 3 g/dL	**24h urine protein > 3.5 g** • nephrotic syndrome **LFTs abnormal** • hepatic failure **prealbumin < 20 mg/dL** • malnutrition
thyroid function tests	**high TSH** • myxedema

B) REGIONAL:

upper extremity	**jugular vein pressure elevated** • superior vena cava syndrome **Doppler or venography** • venous thrombosis • lymphatic obstruction
lower extremity	**Doppler or venogram** • venous thrombosis • lymphatic obstruction

1.43.) EOSINOPHILIA

(> 500/mm^3)

allergy	• drugs • hay fever • asthma
skin disorders	• atopic dermatitis • pemphigus vulgaris
parasites	• trichinosis • toxocara • echinococcus
CXR: pulmonary infiltrate	• Löffler's syndrome [1] (eosinophilic pneumonia)

[1] *eosinophils also found in sputum*

 Eosinophilia is more likely if tissue is invaded by parasites (e.g. trichinosis) than when parasites inhabit the visceral lumen (e.g. tapeworm).

1.44.) EPISTAXIS

local causes	• trauma to Little's area [1] • nasal fracture • nasal tumors • septal granulomas/perforations
systemic cause	• hypertension • coagulopathy • hereditary telangiectasis

[1] *most common cause in children*

 It is important to identify the site of bleeding as accurately as possible in case a vessel needs to be tied later.

1.45.) RED EYE

	ACUTE GLAUCOMA	CONJUNCTIVITIS	UVEITIS	KERATITIS
conjunctiva	conjunctival and ciliary vessels injected	conjunctival vessels injected	ciliary vessels injected	conjunctival vessels injected
		most marked away from corneoscleral margin	most marked on corneoscleral margin	most marked on corneoscleral margin
cornea	hazy, insensitive	clear, sensitive	clear, sensitive	opaque, diminished reflex
iris	injected	normal	swollen, adheres to lens	normal
anterior chamber	shallow	normal	may be turbid	normal
pupil	dilated, fixed	normal	small, fixed	normal
intraocular pressure	increased	normal	normal	normal

1.46.) FATIGUE

1. Check electrolytes and CBC
- anemia
- hypokalemia
- uremia
- diabetes mellitus
- adrenal insufficiency

2. Check for signs of infection
- viral prodrome

chronic infections
- tuberculosis
- endocarditis
- parasitic/fungal

3. Screen for drugs and toxins
- heavy metals
- carbon monoxide
- solvents

4. Perform thyroid tests
- hypothyroidism / hyperthyroidism

5. Search for occult malignancies

6. If none of the above, consider:
- nutritional deficiency
- depression
- severe stress
- chronic fatigue syndrome

1.47.) FEVER

CXR	• tuberculosis • lymphoma
blood, urine, throat cultures	• endocarditis • sepsis • etc…
HIV antibody test	• AIDS
liver function tests	• hepatitis
serology	• Lyme disease • salmonella • typhus • psittacosis
RBC thick smear	• malaria
ESR elevated	• SLE • vasculitis • Still's disease
echocardiogram	• endocarditis • pericarditis
bone scan	• metastatic disease • osteomyelitis
abdominal/pelvic CT scan	• abscess • lymphoma • occult malignancies
viral cultures (expensive, low yield)	• Epstein-Barr virus • cytomegalovirus

1.48.) <u>FOLIC ACID DEFICIENCY</u>
(< 2 ng/mL)

inadequate intake	• alcoholics • infants
impaired absorption	• steatorrhea • sprue • jejunal resection • Whipple's disease • amyloidosis
increased requirements	• pregnancy • infancy • hyperthyroidism • malignancy
impaired metabolism	<u>anti-folates</u>: ➢ pyrimethamine ➢ trimethoprim ➢ methotrexate

1.49.) GAIT ABNORMALITIES

cerebellar	wide base swaying of trunk difficulty walking line heal to toe • multiple sclerosis • medulloblastoma • cerebellar degeneration (alcoholism)
sensory ataxia	Romberg sign (patient falls when closing eyes) patient stomps feet patient watches feet and ground closely • damage to posterior roots/columns • tabes dorsalis • vit. B12 deficiency • multiple sclerosis
labyrinthine	can't focus vision when moving must stop to read signs
Parkinson	involuntary acceleration rigid, shuffling "patient chases his center of gravity"
equine gait (foot drop)	excessive hip flexion to compensate • peroneal nerve damage • poliomyelitis • Charcot-Marie-Tooth disease • (peroneal muscle atrophy)
waddling gait	failure to stabilize weight bearing hip • weakness of gluteal muscles • muscular dystrophy
drunken gait	reels and swamps in many directions apparently unconcerned
hysterical gait	"stiff leg" exaggerated, dystonic posturing

1.50.) <u>GASTROINTESTINAL BLEEDING</u>

hematemesis	**upper GI endoscopy** • esophageal varices • Mallory-Weiss tear • gastric ulcer • duodenal ulcer
hematochezia / melena	**upper GI endoscopy** (as above) **colonoscopy** • infectious colitis • inflammatory bowel disease • neoplasms • ischemic bowel **angiography** • neoplasms • angiodysplasia (malformation)
bright red blood per rectum	**hemorrhoids** • fissures **sigmoidoscopy then colonoscopy** • infectious colitis • inflammatory bowel disease • neoplasms • diverticulitis
occult blood	**evaluate hematocrit and iron** **colonoscopy** **upper GI endoscopy**

1.51.) GYNECOMASTIA

neonatal	**physiologic** • 70% of male neonates • placental estrogens • hCG stimulation of Leydig cells
puberty	**physiologic** (often one-sided) • constitutional sensitivity to estrogen **pathologic** • testicular feminization (androgen insensitivity)
adults	**drugs** ➤ spironolactone ➤ cimetidine ➤ marijuana **pathologic** • bronchogenic carcinoma (ectopic hCG production) • liver disease (reduced estradiol metabolism) • Leydig cell tumor ○ carcinoma of male breast
elderly	**physiologic** ○ decreased testosterone (imbalance in ratio of free testosterone and free estrogen)

1.52.) <u>ACUTE HEADACHE</u>

A) <u>SUDDEN ONSET</u>:

recent trauma	no focal signs → observe focal signs → MRI • subdural hemorrhage
no trauma	MRI • subarachnoid hemorrhage

B) <u>GRADUAL ONSET</u>:

history of trauma	MRI scan • subdural hemorrhage
fever plus nuchal rigidity or fever plus focal signs	lumbar puncture • meningitis • encephalitis
no fever	MRI scan • tumors • brain abscess • intracranial bleed

1.53.) CHRONIC HEADACHE

unilateral, throbbing	**aura** • classic migraine [1] **no aura** • common migraine [1]
unilateral, non-throbbing	**lacrimation, rhinorrhea** • cluster headache **tender temporal artery** • temporal arteritis
bilateral, non-throbbing	• tension headache
other	• hypertensive headache

[1] *may also be bilateral and throbbing*

Consider temporal arteritis in all patients >50 years. Early diagnosis prevents visual loss.

1.54.) HEARING LOSS

conductive deafness	**Weber test: lateralized to sick ear** **Rinne test: negative (can't hear)** • occlusion of external auditory canal • cholesteatoma • chronic otitis • otosclerosis
nerve deafness	**Weber test: lateralized to healthy ear** **Rinne test: positive (can hear)** • cochlear disease • cochlear nerve damage
central deafness	**brainstem evoked auditory potentials (BAEP)** • damage to cochlear nuclei

Weber test: *Place tuning fork on top of skull.*
Rinne test: *Place tuning fork on mastoid process. When sound ceases, hold next to auditory meatus (should be able to hear again).*

BAEP is a very sensitive measure to detect acoustic neuromas or other tumors of cerebellopontine angle.

1.55.) HEMATURIA

a/w white cell casts	• pyelonephritis
a/w red cell casts	• SLE • chronic glomerulonephritis
urine culture	• cystitis • pyelonephritis • prostatitis • TB
urine protein < 1 g/24h	**IVP or cystoscopy** • tumor, cyst, stones • papillary necrosis • cystitis **renal arteriogram** • AV-malformation • renal infarction • tumors
urine protein > 1 g/24h	**if renal biopsy abnormal:** • glomerulonephritis • interstitial nephritis • vasculitis **if renal biopsy unremarkable:** • benign familial hematuria • runner's hematuria

Cystoscopy has ~90% sensitivity to detect bladder cancer.
Urine cytology has ~70% sensitivity to detect bladder cancer.

1.56.) HEMOPTYSIS

1. Get coagulation workup
- coagulopathy
- thrombocytopenia
- leukemia

2. Chest X-ray → solitary lesion
- carcinoma
- granuloma
- bronchogenic cyst

Chest X-ray → diffuse infiltrate
if culture positive:
- bacterial, fungal, parasitic

if culture negative:
- pulmonary sequestration
- hemorrhagic telangiectasis

3. Check ECG for valvular disease
- mitral stenosis / pulmonic stenosis

4. Consider bronchoscopy
- bronchitis
- neoplasm
- foreign body

5. Consider pulmonary angiogram:
- pulmonary embolus / infarction
- AV fistula

1.57.) HEPATOMEGALY

1. Get serology
- HAV, HBV, HCV
- cytomegalovirus

↓

2. Increased central vein pressure?
- congestive heart failure
- constrictive pericarditis
- tricuspid regurgitation

↓

3. Get CT or MRI scan
- cysts (echinococcus etc.)
- hepatocellular carcinoma
- metastases

↓

4. Consider liver biopsy
- toxic or alcoholic hepatitis
- α1-antitrypsin deficiency
- Wilson's disease
- Gaucher's disease
- lymphoma

↓

5. Consider venogram:
- Budd-Chiari syndrome
  (obstruction of hepatic veins)

1.58.) HIRSUTISM

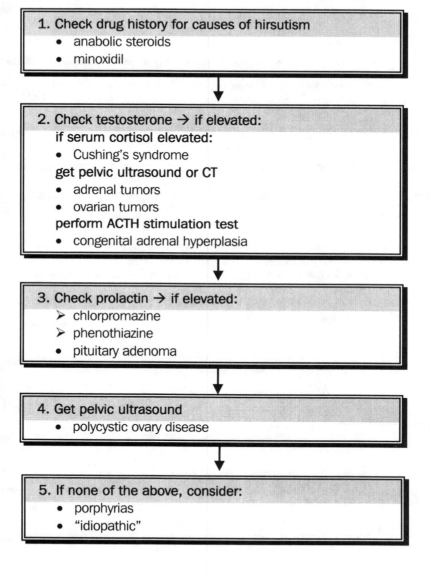

1. Check drug history for causes of hirsutism
- anabolic steroids
- minoxidil

2. Check testosterone → if elevated:
if serum cortisol elevated:
- Cushing's syndrome

get pelvic ultrasound or CT
- adrenal tumors
- ovarian tumors

perform ACTH stimulation test
- congenital adrenal hyperplasia

3. Check prolactin → if elevated:
- ➢ chlorpromazine
- ➢ phenothiazine
- pituitary adenoma

4. Get pelvic ultrasound
- polycystic ovary disease

5. If none of the above, consider:
- porphyrias
- "idiopathic"

1.59.) HYPERCALCEMIA
(Ca^{2+} > 10 mg/dL)

albumin > 5.2 g/dL	**ionized calcium normal:** • pseudohypercalcemia
drugs	➢ thiazide diuretics
PTH elevated	**primary hyperparathyroidism:** • parathyroid adenoma • MEN 1 • MEN 2 **secondary hyperparathyroidism:** • renal failure • malabsorption
vit. D elevated	• vit. D intoxication
other	**increased bone release:** • immobilization • malignancy • milk-alkali syndrome

1.60.) HYPERCAPNIA

(CO_2 > 45 mm Hg)

chest trauma	• flail chest • airway obstruction
pH > 7.4	metabolic alkalosis with respiratory compensation
HCO_3 > 29 mM/L	chronic respiratory acidosis • COPD • interstitial lung disease • kyphoscoliosis • polio • amyotrophic lateral sclerosis • muscular dystrophy
CXR	parenchymal lung disease • pneumonia • ARDS • pulmonary edema • pulmonary embolus
low expiratory pressure	neuromuscular weakness • botulism • Guillain-Barré syndrome • myasthenia gravis
low FEV_1	obstructive disease • asthma • bronchospasm
other	○ drugs ○ loss of respiratory drive (CNS) [1]

[1] *Do NOT give 100% O_2 to patients with chronic hypoxia !*

1.61.) HYPERKALEMIA
(K$^+$ > 5.5 mM/L)

WBC > 100,000 or platelets > 1,000,000	**pseudohyperkalemia** • leukocytosis • thrombocytosis
drugs	➤ digitalis ➤ ACE inhibitors ➤ K sparing diuretics
urine K$^+$ > 20 mM/L	**increased K$^+$ load** • dietary • GI bleeding • massive blood transfusion **transcellular shift** • acidosis • hyperglycemia/insulin deficiency **CPK or uric acid elevated** • rhabdomyolysis • tumor lysis
urine K$^+$ < 20 mM/L	**low aldosterone** • hypoaldosteronism **high creatinine** • renal failure **defective tubular K$^+$ secretion** • obstructive nephropathy • amyloidosis • SLE

1.62.) HYPERLIPIDEMIA

(triglycerides > 250 mg/dL)
(cholesterol > 200 mg/dL)

triglycerides high cholesterol normal	primary hyperlipidemia type I **secondary** • diabetes
cholesterol high triglycerides normal	primary hyperlipidemia type IIa **secondary** • renal failure • liver disease • porphyria
cholesterol high **triglycerides high**	primary hyperlipidemia **secondary** • diabetes mellitus • nephrotic syndrome • Cushing's syndrome

1.63.) HYPERNATREMIA
(Na$^+$ > 145 mM/L)

> **1. Assess volume status:**
> * pulse, skin turgor, mucous membranes

hypovolemia	**urine Na$^+$ < 10 mM/L** • diarrhea • sweating **urine Na$^+$ > 20 mM/L** • osmotic diuresis ➤ diuretics
volume normal	**urine osmolarity high** • respiratory loss • skin loss **urine osmolarity low** • central diabetes insipidus • renal diabetes insipidus
hypervolemia	**iatrogenic hypernatremia** ➤ hypertonic saline ➤ hypertonic NaHCO$_3$

1.64.) HYPERPHOSPHATEMIA
(PO$_4$ > 5 mg/dL)

A) IF URINE PHOSPHATE > 1,500 mg/24h:

increased cell turnover (CPK, LDH, uric acid elevated)	• hemolysis • leukemia • tumor lysis • rhabdomyolysis
increased load	• transfusion of stored blood • vit. D intoxication
redistribution	• acidosis • hyperglycemia/insulin deficiency

B) IF URINE PHOSPHATE < 1,500 mg/24h:

creatinine clearance < 25 mL/min	• renal failure
Ca^{2+} < 8.5 mg/dL	**PTH low** • hypoparathyroidism **PTH normal** • pseudohypoparathyroidism
other	• hyperthyroidism • tumor calcinosis

 Decreased renal clearance is the most common cause of hyperphosphatemia.

1.65.) HYPERTENSION

A) GENERAL WORKUP:

> **1. Check drug history for causes of hypertension**
> - oral contraceptives
>
> - sympathomimetics
> - cocaine
>
> - glucocorticoids
> - mineralocorticoids

2. If K^+ < 3.5 mM/L:
check plasma renin → if low:
- primary hyperaldosteronism

B) IF AGE OF ONSET > 30 YEARS:

1. Therapeutic trial → if adequate control:
- most likely "essential hypertension"

2. Therapeutic trial → if inadequate control:
- evaluate for secondary hypertension
  (see next)

B) IF AGE OF ONSET < 30 YEARS
  evaluate for secondary hypertension:

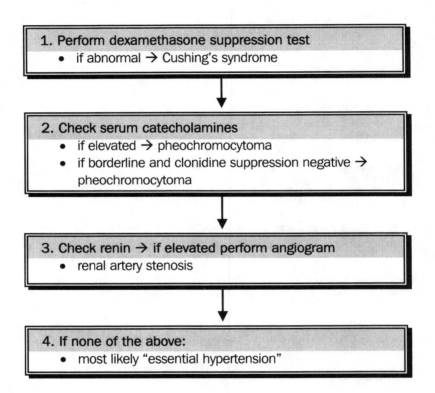

1. Perform dexamethasone suppression test
   - if abnormal → Cushing's syndrome

2. Check serum catecholamines
   - if elevated → pheochromocytoma
   - if borderline and clonidine suppression negative → pheochromocytoma

3. Check renin → if elevated perform angiogram
   - renal artery stenosis

4. If none of the above:
   - most likely "essential hypertension"

1.66.) HYPOCALCEMIA
(Ca^{2+} < 8.4 mg/dL)

albumin < 4 g/dL	**ionized Ca^{2+} normal** • reduction in protein bound Ca^{2+} only
low PTH	• hypoparathyroidism (head and neck surgery)
low phosphate low vit. D	**decreased Ca^{2+} intake** • nutritional deficiency • malabsorption **decreased vit. D production** • renal disease • liver disease • rickets • pseudohypoparathyroidism
other	o acute pancreatitis o hyperphosphatemia

1.67.) <u>HYPOGLYCEMIA</u>
(< 50 mg/dL)

drugs	➢ insulin ➢ sulfonylureas ➢ beta-blockers
food tolerance test	**postprandial hypoglycemia** • early diabetes mellitus • dumping syndrome • "idiopathic"
72h fast: low glucose, high insulin	**elevated C-peptide** • insulinoma **low C-peptide** • insulin (factitious) • insulin antibodies
72h fast: high glucose, low insulin	**insulin resistance** • obesity • polycystic ovary disease • pregnancy
other	**artifact** • leukocytosis etc. [1]

[1] *low glucose levels in whole blood, but normal in serum.*

1.68.) HYPOKALEMIA
(K^+ < 3.5 mM/L)

drugs	➤ diuretics
urine K^+ > 20 mM/L	**ELEVATED BLOOD PRESSURE:** **high renin** • renal artery stenosis • malignant hypertension • renin-secreting tumors **low renin** • hyperaldosteronism • Cushing's syndrome **METABOLIC ACIDOSIS:** • renal tubular acidosis **METABOLIC ALKALOSIS:** **urine Cl^- < 10 mM/L** • vomiting **urine Cl^- > 20 mM/L** • Bartter's syndrome • osmotic diuresis
urine K^+ variable	**increased cell uptake** • leukemia • insulin
urine K^+ < 20 mM/L	**decreased intake** • starvation, anorexia **GI loss** • laxatives, diarrhea

1.69.) HYPONATREMIA
(Na⁺ < 135 mM/L)

serum osmolality >295 mosm/kg	**pseudohyponatremia** • hyperglycemia • hyperlipidemia
edema (total body Na⁺ increased)	**urine Na⁺ >20 mM/L** • renal failure **urine Na⁺ <10 mM/L** • congestive heart failure • nephrotic syndrome • cirrhosis

dehydration
(total body Na⁺ decreased)
	urine Na⁺ >20 mM/L
	• renal loss
	  - diuretic excess
	  - osmotic diuresis
	  - ketonuria
	• adrenal insufficiency
	
	urine Na⁺ <10 mM/L
	• GI loss
	• third space loss

other	○ psychogenic polydipsia • SIADH [1] • CNS lesions • small cell carcinoma • non-malignant pulmonary diseases

[1] *severe pain, nausea and stress also stimulate ADH release*

1.70.) <u>HYPOPHOSPHATEMIA</u>
(PO$_4$ < 2.5 mg/dL)

intracellular/extracellular shift	• alkalosis ➤ insulin
urine PO$_4$ < 100 mg/24h	**decreased intake** • alcoholism • malabsorption • phosphate binders • vit. D deficiency
urine PO$_4$ > 100 mg/24h	**hyperparathyroidism** **tubular defects** • Fanconi syndrome • vit. D resistant rickets ➤ diuretics

1.71.) <u>HYPOTENSION</u>

A) <u>ORTHOSTATIC HYPOTENSION</u>:

intravascular volume decreased	blood loss dehydration adrenal insufficiency shock • anaphylactic • septic • toxic shock syndrome third space loss of fluid • ascites • pleural effusion • edema
drugs	➤ diuretics ➤ calcium channel blockers ➤ nitroglycerin ➤ phenothiazines ➤ tricyclic antidepressants

B) <u>NON-ORTHOSTATIC HYPOTENSION</u>:

pale, sweating	• vasovagal hypotension
cardiovascular signs	• heart failure • valvular disease • pericardial tamponade • arrhythmia
intravascular volume decreased	(see above)

1.72.) <u>URINARY INCONTINENCE</u>

stress incontinence (coughing, strain)	**voiding cystourethrogram** • urethral hypermobility (90%) • damaged internal sphincter (10%)
urge incontinence "uninhibited bladder"	**urinalysis / culture** • bacterial cystitis **cystoscopy** • bladder tumor • urethral obstruction (prostate !)
overflow incontinence	• diabetic neuropathy • multiple sclerosis **drugs** ➢ anticholinergics
other	• fistulae: continuous incontinence

1.73.) <u>INSOMNIA</u>

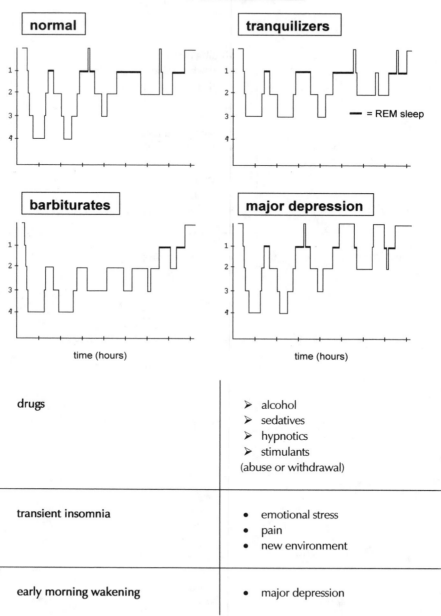

drugs	➢ alcohol ➢ sedatives ➢ hypnotics ➢ stimulants (abuse or withdrawal)
transient insomnia	• emotional stress • pain • new environment
early morning wakening	• major depression

1.74.) JAUNDICE - I

A) UNCONJUGATED BILIRUBIN > 0.4 mg/dL

hereditary	**transferase deficiency** • Gilbert's syndrome • Crigler-Najjar syndrome
neonatal	**immature transferase**
drugs	**acquired transferase deficiency** ➢ chloramphenicol ➢ pregnanediol
hematocrit < 38	• hemolytic anemia
no evidence of hemolysis	• lipid-poor hyperalimentation

 In most hepatocellular diseases, bilirubin excretion is more impaired than bilirubin conjugation.
(➔ conjugated hyperbilirubinemia is more common)

1.75.) JAUNDICE - II

B) CONJUGATED BILIRUBIN > 0.4 mg/dL

drugs	➢ oral contraceptives ➢ chlorpromazine ➢ erythromycin ➢ isoniazid ➢ halothane ➢ phenytoin
alk. phosphatase > 300 U/L	**ultrasound: dilated bile duct** • stones • sclerosing cholangitis • pancreatic tumor **CT scan / MRI** • cirrhosis • tumor metastasis • granulomas **other** • viral hepatitis • primary biliary cirrhosis
ALT or AST > 300 U/L	**viral serologies** • viral hepatitis **liver biopsy** • toxic hepatitis • alcoholic hepatitis • infiltrative disease • primary biliary cirrhosis
ALT or AST < 300 U/L	• Dubin-Johnson syndrome • Rotor syndrome

1.76.) <u>LOWER BACK PAIN</u>

1. Get skeletal X-ray series
- osteoarthritis
- compression fracture
- ankylosing spondylitis

bone diseases:
- osteomalacia
- osteoporosis

2. Get CT or MRI scan:
- spinal tumors
- disc herniation
- vertebral compression fracture

3. Abnormal physical exam (imaging normal)
- pancreatitis
- lumbosacral strain

4. ESR elevated (imaging normal)
- polymyalgia rheumatica

5. If none of the above, consider:
- malingering

1.77.) LYMPHADENOPATHY

A) GENERALIZED:

CBC abnormal	• lymphoma • leukemia
CBC variable	• connective tissue diseases **infections:** • AIDS • TB • syphilis
CBC normal	• Whipple's disease • sarcoidosis • lipid storage disease

B) LOCALIZED:

head/neck	• head/neck cancer • lymphoma
supraclavicular	• lung cancer • stomach cancer • breast cancer
axillary	• breast cancer • lung cancer
inguinal	• rectal cancer • prostate cancer • gynecological cancer
biopsy negative	**local inflammation:** • Kawasaki's disease

80

1.78.) LYMPHOCYTOSIS
(> 4,000/mm^3)

atypical lymphocytes	**heterophile ab test positive:** • mononucleosis (EBV) **heterophile ab test negative:** • mononucleosis (CMV) • hepatitis
lymphadenopathy **splenomegaly**	• infections • leukemia • lymphoma
bone marrow biopsy	• ALL • CLL • hairy cell leukemia • multiple myeloma • non-Hodgkin's lymphoma
other	• viral infections • pertussis • tuberculosis • syphilis

Viral infections more commonly than bacterial infections cause lymphocytosis.

1.79.) METROMENORRHAGIA

(excessive, irregular bleeding)

---

1. Perform pelvic exam
irregular uterus:
- myoma

symmetrically enlarged uterus:
- adenomyosis
- endometrial carcinoma

↓

2. Cytologic exam:
Not reliable for diagnosis of endometrial abnormalities.
However, women in secretory phase of menstrual cycle
should not shed endometrial cells.
- if abnormal → further evaluation required

↓

3. perform D&C – "gold standard" for diagnosis of:
- endometrial hyperplasia vs. carcinoma

Vabra aspirator or pipelle sampler:
- easier and painless compared to D&C
- has become method of choice

---

*Most women have occasional menstrual cycles that are not in
their usual pattern. Just observe!*

DYSFUNCTIONAL UTERINE BLEEDING:
Bleeding from proliferative endometrium as a result of
anovulation in the absence of organic disease.

Recommended workup: Pap smear
                        pregnancy test
                        CBC
                        endometrial biopsy.

1.80.) <u>MONOCYTOSIS</u>
(> 750/mm³)

abnormal CBC

diagnostic bone marrow:
- myeloid metaplasia
- leukemia
- multiple myeloma
- preleukemia
- lymphoma

other:
- malignant histiocytosis
- polycythemia vera
- ITP

variable CBC

infections:
- tuberculosis [1]
- mononucleosis

- sarcoidosis
- autoimmune diseases

[1] *poor prognostic sign if monocytosis develops*

Infectious disease is an uncommon cause of monocytosis. More than 50% are associated with hematologic disease.

1.81.) <u>MUSCLE WEAKNESS</u>

1. Perform neurological exam
- Guillain-Barré syndrome
- amyotrophic lateral sclerosis
- myasthenia gravis
- porphyria

2. Check electrolytes and metabolic abnormalities
- hypo/hyperkalemia
- hypo/hyperthyroidism
- hypercalcemia
- Cushing's syndrome
- ○ familial periodic paralysis
- ○ familial myoglobinuria

3. Creatine kinase elevated?
EMG abnormal:
- polymyositis
- dermatomyositis
muscle biopsy abnormal:
- muscular dystrophy

4. ESR elevated?
- polymyalgia rheumatica
- rheumatoid arthritis
- polyarteritis nodosa
- SLE

5. If none of the above, consider:
- depression

1.82.) <u>NEUTROPENIA</u>
(< 1,500/mm^3)

drugs	**antibiotics** ➤ sulfonamides ➤ penicillins ➤ antihistamines ➤ indomethacin ➤ phenothiazines ➤ propylthiouracil ➤ oral hypoglycemics
infections	• sepsis • viral, bacterial, parasitic
splenomegaly	• hypersplenism
bone marrow biopsy	• myelodysplastic syndromes • myelophthisic syndromes • acute leukemia

1.83.) NEUTROPHILIA

$(> 10,000/mm^3)$

drugs	➢ lithium ➢ digoxin
reactive neutrophilia	• infections • inflammations
bone marrow biopsy	• AML • CML • myelofibrosis • polycythemia vera
other	○ post-splenectomy ○ stress ○ "idiopathic"

1.84.) NIPPLE DISCHARGE

clear or serous **from multiple ducts**	➤ oral contraceptives
unilateral **from single duct**	• usually intraductal papilloma • rarely intraductal carcinoma
prior to menstruation **unilateral or bilateral**	• usually fibrocystic change
milky (increased prolactin)	**drugs** ➤ phenothiazines ➤ methyldopa **CNS lesions** • "empty sella" • pituitary adenoma • hypothalamic tumor

 Cytologic exam of nipple discharge is specific but not sensitive.
(i.e. negative result does not exclude carcinoma)

 If unilateral discharge persists → need to explore further.

1.85.) <u>OLIGURIA - I</u>
(< 400 mL/day)

A) U_{Na} < 20 mM/L, FE_{Na} < 1

prerenal failure	hypovolemia
	• shock
	• blood loss
	• third-space loss of fluid
	• heart failure
	renal vascular resistance
	• malignant hypertension
	• toxemia of pregnancy
	• thrombosis
	• hepatorenal syndrome
nephritic sediment	• acute glomerulonephritis

 Prerenal failure causes 80% of oliguria.

FRACTIONAL EXCRETION OF SODIUM:

Divide Na excretion by creatinine excretion:

$$FE_{Na} = (U_{Na} / P_{Na}) / (U_{cr} / P_{cr})$$

1.86.) OLIGURIA - II

B) $U_{Na} > 20$ mM/L, $FE_{Na} > 2$

---

1. Check urine protein, if >1 g/24h:
nephritic sediment:
- chronic glomerulonephritis

non-nephritic sediment:
- vasculitis

---

2. Get renal ultrasound
postrenal failure
- stones
- neoplasms
- papillary debris
- prostatic hypertrophy
- congenital urethral obstruction

---

3. Consider gallium scan, if abnormal:
interstitial nephritis
- eosinophils → allergic
- no eosinophils → infection

---

4. If none of the above, consider:
ATN
- ischemic
- toxic

1.87.) PANCYTOPENIA

MARROW: hypocellular	**marrow infiltration** • lymphoma • multiple myeloma • TB, sarcoid, fungi • myelofibrosis **aplastic anemia** • toxins • Fanconi
MARROW: normal or hypercellular	• myelodysplasia ○ B_{12} deficiency ○ folate deficiency ○ hypersplenism ○ AIDS
other	○ overwhelming infection

1.88.) PARALYSIS

particular muscle group	• **peripheral nerve damage** a/w typical sensory deficits severe atrophy if complete denervation
monoplegia	• **hysterical paralysis** characteristic gait: "stiff leg" tendon reflexes present atrophy absent • **multiple sclerosis** spasticity → UMN atrophy → LMN
hemiplegia	• **cortical or subcortical lesion** a/w aphasia, astereognosis etc. • **brainstem lesion** a/w eye or tongue motor dysfunction • **Brown-Séquard syndrome** a/w contralateral loss of pain/temperature

paraplegia
(thoracolumbar cord)
tetraplegia
(cervical cord)
	ACUTE:
	spinal cord trauma
	
	SLOWLY PROGRESSING:
	children: muscular dystrophy
	            Friedreich's ataxia
	
	adults: multiple sclerosis
	         vit. B12 deficiency
	         spinal tumors
	         syringomyelia

1.89.) PLEURAL EFFUSION

cardiac exam	• congestive heart failure
thoracocentesis : transudate	• congestive heart failure • cirrhosis • nephrotic syndrome • hypoalbuminemia
thoracocentesis : exudate	**cytology positive** • malignancy **mononuclear cells** • tuberculosis • viral infection **polymorphonuclear cells** • bacterial infection **amylase > 200 U/dL** • pancreatitis **ANA positive** • SLE **miscellaneous** o drug reaction o uremia o pericardial disease
thoracocentesis : blood	• trauma • malignancy • pulmonary infarction

1.90.) <u>POLYCYTHEMIA</u>

1. Rule out pseudopolycythemia
- dehydration

2. Check arterial O_2 saturation, if <90%:
altitude
lung disease
- pulmonary AV fistula
- COPD
- interstitial fibrosis
- hypoventilation

congenital heart disease
- R→L shunt

3. Check erythropoietin level, if elevated:
Kidney diseases
- hydronephrosis
- polycystic kidney disease
- adenoma
- hypernephroma

Liver tumors

Get hemoglobin electrophoresis:
- abnormal hemoglobins
- methemoglobin
- carboxyhemoglobin

4. If erythropoietin is normal:
- polycythemia vera

1.91.) POLYURIA

(> 3 L/day)

A) <u>Polyuria due to solute load</u>: urine > 300 mosm/L

> **1. Search for cause**
> - diabetes mellitus
> - chronic renal failure
> - diuretic therapy

B) <u>Polyuria due to water diuresis</u>: urine < 300 mosm/L

> **1. Water deprivation → if urine concentrates:**
> - psychogenic polydipsia

↓

> **2. Water deprivation → if urine does not concentrate:**
> - diabetes insipidus

↓

> **3. Give vasopressin**
> **if urine concentrates → cranial causes**
> - empty sella
> - sella tumor
> - Sheehan's syndrome
>
> **if urine does not concentrate → renal causes**
> - nephrotoxins
> - any severe chronic renal disease

94

1.92.) PROTEINURIA

(> 150 mg/24h)

urine protein < 3 g/24h	**URINE PROTEIN ELECTROPHORESIS:** **light chains** [1] • multiple myeloma **albumin only** • minimal change GN • transient (exercise, fever) **beta microglobulin** • tubular injury
urine protein > 3 g/24h	**genetic diseases** • Alport's syndrome • Fabry's disease • sickle cell anemia **renal biopsy → kidney disease** • glomerulonephritis **renal biopsy → systemic disease** • malignant hypertension • SLE • Goodpasture's syndrome • Henoch-Schönlein purpura • amyloidosis

[1] *urine dip stick false negative! (light chains do not react chemically)*

SERUM BETA MICROGLOBULIN	URINE BETA MICROGLOBULIN
glomerular disease - diabetic nephropathy - transplant rejection	**tubular injury** - interstitial nephritis - ATN - toxins

1.93.) PRURITUS

1. Characteristic skin lesions present?
- atopic dermatitis
- allergic dermatitis

- urticaria
- folliculitis
- pemphigoid
- psoriasis
- mycosis fungoides

- lichen simplex chronicus

2. Check drug history
- hypersensitivity reaction
- amphetamines

3. Lymph nodes enlarged?
- lymphoma

4. Dysproteinemia?
- multiple myeloma

5. Abnormal liver function tests?
- obstructive biliary disease

6. elevated BUN / creatinine?
- uremia

1.94.) PURPURA

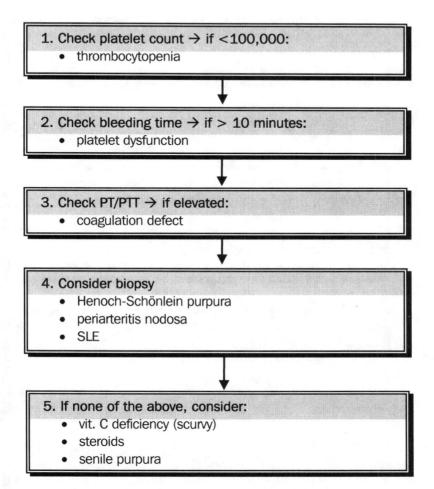

1. Check platelet count → if <100,000:
- thrombocytopenia

2. Check bleeding time → if > 10 minutes:
- platelet dysfunction

3. Check PT/PTT → if elevated:
- coagulation defect

4. Consider biopsy
- Henoch-Schönlein purpura
- periarteritis nodosa
- SLE

5. If none of the above, consider:
- vit. C deficiency (scurvy)
- steroids
- senile purpura

1.95.) <u>RIGHT HEART FAILURE</u>

1. Get Chest X-ray and ECG
- inferior myocardial infarction

if cor pulmonale → get pulmonary function test
- obstructive disease (COPD)
- restrictive disease

2. If murmurs are present → get echocardiogram
valvular diseases:
- mitral stenosis
- tricuspid regurgitation
- pulmonary regurgitation
- pulmonary stenosis

3. Consider cardiac catheterization
shunt:
- atrial septal defect
- ventricular septal defect
- patent ductus arteriosus

4. Consider V/Q scan
- pulmonary embolus

5. Consider Swan-Ganz catheter
- primary pulmonary hypertension

1.96.) SCROTAL SWELLING

A) PAINLESS:

hydrocele	tense fluctuant **transilluminates**
varicocele	soft worm-like does not transilluminate **collapses when patient lies down** [1]
spermatocele	vaguely circumscribed does not transilluminate **persists when patient lies down**
tumor	hard insensitive to pressure

[1] *if a "varicocele" does not collapse, suspect retroperitoneal neoplasm.*

B) PAINFUL:

torsion	young boys normal urinalysis → **elevation of scrotum intensifies pain**
epididymitis	more common after puberty pyuria → **elevation of scrotum reduces pain**

1.97.) <u>SEIZURE</u>

1. If there is a history of trauma → get CT or MRI
CT scan abnormal:
- subdural hematoma
- intracranial bleed

CT scan normal:
- concussion

2. Check blood pressure
- hypertensive encephalopathy

3. Search for metabolic disorders and toxins
- hypocalcemia
- hypoglycemia
- hypoxia
➢ alcohol
➢ cocaine
➢ amphetamines

4. Get EEG
- epileptic disorder

5. Get CT or MRI scan
- tumors, infarction, bleeding

6. Fever or nuchal rigidity → do lumbar puncture
- meningitis
- encephalitis

1.98.) <u>SKIN RASH - ADULTS</u>

	RASH	OTHER SYMPTOMS
drug eruptions	- bright red - intensely pruritic	2 days ~ 2 weeks after drug was given
infectious mononucleosis	- diffuse maculopapular	pharyngitis lymphadenopathy hepatosplenomegaly
Lyme disease	- papule, expanding to large annular lesion with central clearing	headache, myalgia photophobia arthritis weeks later
typhoid fever	- "rose spots" (small macules/papules on trunk)	abdominal pain diarrhea
SLE	- erythema in sun-exposed areas - "butterfly rash"	multi-organ disease
2° syphilis	- copper colored, scaly, papular, - on palms and soles	primary chancre coexisting in 10%
erythema nodosum	- large subcutaneous nodules on lower legs - very tender	arthralgia
Rocky Mountain spotted fever	- maculopapular - beginning on wrists and ankle - spreading to trunk	fever, headache myalgia

1.99.) <u>SKIN RASH - CHILDREN</u>

	RASH	OTHER SYMPTOMS
measles (rubeola)	- discrete lesions that become confluent. - spread from hairline down - spare palms and soles	cough conjunctivitis coryza
German measles (rubella)	- spreads from hairline down - clearing while spreading	adenopathy
erythema infectiosum	- bright red - "slapped cheek" appearance	mild fever
exanthema subitum	- diffuse maculopapular - spares face	rash follows resolution of fever
hand-foot-mouth dis. (Coxsackie virus)	- mouth: tender vesicles - hands, feet: papules	fever
scarlet fever	- diffuse blanchable erythema - spread from face to trunk - "sand paper" texture	fever pharyngitis

1.100.) SPLENOMEGALY

CBC, ultrasound	spleen displaced by: • renal mass, ovarian mass etc. • metastases • cysts
congested	• cirrhosis • portal vein thrombosis/compression • congestive heart failure
inflammatory	• SLE • sarcoidosis
infectious	• HIV • mononucleosis • sepsis • parasitic infections
hyperplastic	• hemolytic anemias • TTP
infiltrated	• lymphoma • leukemia • histiocytosis X • lysosomal storage diseases
other	o "idiopathic"

 A palpable spleen is usually an enlarged spleen.

1.101.) <u>STRIDOR - CHILDREN</u>

congenital	choanal atresia
infections	**~2 years old:** croup
	2-7 years old: epiglottitis
	any age: diphtheria
	teenager: infectious mononucleosis

ACUTE EPIGLOTTITIS	ACUTE LARYNGOTRACHEOBRONCHITIS (croup)
• rapid onset • "sore throat" • child appears very ill • child prefers to sit upright • child drools saliva • *H. influenza*	• 1-2 days of upper respiratory infect. • harsh, barking cough • chest wall recessing during inspiration • *parainfluenza virus, RSV, others*

1.102.) <u>STRIDOR - ADULTS</u>

1. Perform external exam
- goiter
- thyroid neoplasm

2. Consider laryngoscopy
- retropharyngeal abscess
- laryngitis
- diphtheria
- injury (post-endotracheal tube)

3. Consider bronchoscopy, biopsy
- narrowing of bronchi
- bronchial carcinoma
- mediastinal tumors
- tuberculosis/sarcoidosis

If stridor occurs after neck surgery, suspect damage to recurrent nerve.

1.103.) <u>SYNCOPE</u>

1. Check electrolytes, glucose, hematocrit...
- adrenal insufficiency
- hypoglycemia
- blood loss
- dehydration

2. Check blood pressure
- orthostatic hypotension

3. Cardiac monitoring
- arrhythmias

4. If EEG shows seizure activity → get CT or MRI
if brain imaging abnormal:
- mass lesion
- hematoma
- AV- malformation

if brain imaging normal:
- epilepsy

5. Attempt carotid sinus massage
- carotid sinus syncope

6. If none of the above, consider:
- vasovagal syncope

 Distinguish from seizure, vertigo and narcolepsy!

1.104.) TACHYCARDIA
(> 100 beats/min)

sinus tachycardia	**physiologic response** • (exercise, stress, hypotension etc.)
atrial fibrillation	• fever • congestive heart failure • thyrotoxicosis
atrial flutter	• organic heart diseases
ventricular preexcitation (WPW)	• AV bypass tracts (strands of atrial muscle around AV ring)
ventricular tachycardia	• chronic ischemia • prior MI • cardiomyopathy • drug toxicity
ventricular flutter/fibrillation	• ischemic heart disease

WPW: Catheter ablation of bypass tract successful in 90% of cases (recommended for symptomatic and asymptomatic patients).

1.105.) <u>THROMBOCYTOPENIA</u>

(< 150,000 mm^3)

CBC	**"artifact"** • platelet clumps
bone marrow: **(low megakaryocytes)**	**defective maturation:** • B12 deficiency • folate deficiency • iron deficiency **decreased thrombocytopoiesis:** • drugs • radiation • aplastic anemia • myelofibrosis - lymphoma/leukemia
bone marrow: **(normal or high megakaryocytes)**	**myelodysplastic syndromes** **hereditary** • Wiskott-Aldrich

	PERIPHERAL DESTRUCTION:
	• splenomegaly
	
	• immunological
	   - ITP
	   - sensitization (prior transfusions)

	PERIPHERAL CONSUMPTION: • DIC • TTP • hemolytic-uremic syndrome • prosthetic valves

1.106.) THROMBOCYTOSIS
(> 400,000 mm^3)

> 1,000,000 platelets no other abnormalities	"primary" thrombocythemia
bone marrow abnormal	myeloproliferative disorders: • polycythemia vera • multiple myeloma • CML • myelofibrosis
bone marrow reactive	• inflammatory diseases • infectious diseases • acute hemorrhage • carcinomas • lymphomas
other	o stress o exercise

1.107.) THYROID ENLARGEMENT

goitrogens	➤ lithium ➤ iodine ➤ kelp
low TSH **high free T4, T3**	**radioactive iodine uptake high:** • Jod Basedow • thyroid carcinoma • Graves' disease [1] • Plummer's disease [2] **radioactive iodine uptake low:** • struma ovarii • thyroiditis
high TSH **low free T4, T3**	• endemic goiter • Hashimoto's • lithium
high TSH **high free T4, T3**	• pituitary adenoma

[1] *diffuse toxic goiter*
[2] *multinodular toxic goiter*

1.108.) THYROID NODULE

fine needle aspiration: diagnostic	• adenoma • cyst • papillary carcinoma • follicular carcinoma • medullary carcinoma
fine needle aspiration: non-diagnostic	THYROID SCAN: cold nodule • repeat needle aspiration or biopsy hot nodule • thyroid adenoma • colloid adenoma

Solitary nodules can be found in 5% of adults.
Most are benign adenomas.

Hot nodules: >99% benign
Cold nodules: 90% benign

Increased risk of malignancy: male
                                 hoarseness
                                 history of neck radiation

1.109.) <u>TINNITUS</u>

"crackling" noise	• cerumen • foreign body in auditory meatus
"bubbling" noise	• middle ear inflammation • otosclerosis
"pulsatile" noise	• internal carotid artery thrombosis • hypertension
"high pitch" noise	**cochlear damage:** • exposure to excessive noise • Ménière's disease [1] • fracture of base of skull **drugs:** ➤ aminoglycosides ➤ quinine

[1] *tinnitus, recurrent vertigo, progressive deafness*

 Prominent tinnitus is often the first symptom of otosclerosis!

1.110.) <u>TRANSAMINASES</u>
(normal 0-35 U/L AST, ALT)

ELEVATED:

history of ethanol	• ask to refrain, then repeat
drugs	• oral contraceptives • acetaminophen • heparin • other toxins
bilirubin high **alkaline phosphatase high**	• cholestasis
CPK high	**cerebral infarction** **acute muscle injury** • IM injections • severe exercise • polymyositis • acute myocardial infarction
liver biopsy	**acute hepatocellular disease** • viral hepatitis • infiltrative diseases • drugs • toxins • alcohol

> **Transaminase level:** viral hepatitis > toxic > alcoholic > tumors

1.111.) <u>TREMOR</u>

physiological tremor	10 Hz (enhanced by isometric muscle contraction)
enhanced physiological tremor	anxiety exercise caffeine alcohol withdrawal
Parkinson	coarse, 3-5 Hz at rest forearms, hands, "pill-rolling" **suppressed during muscle activity** [1]
ataxic tremor (intention tremor) [2]	cerebellar disease **strongest during precise, exacting movements**
familial tremor	less coarse than Parkinson's adult onset head and hands relieved by small amounts of alcohol [3]

[1] *These patients can raise a full glass of water and drink its content without spilling a drop.*

[2] *Does not occur when movement is "intended" but rather when approaching intended target.*

[3] *These patients are often mistaken for alcoholics by the layperson.*

114

1.112.) URTICARIA

1. If acute (< 6 weeks) consider:
atopic condition
- contact urticaria
- food allergy
- drug allergy

- transfusion reactions
- serum sickness

↓

2. Check CBC, ANA etc.
autoimmune diseases
- SLE
- connective tissue diseases

↓

3. Consider biopsy
- angioedema
- vasculitis
- bullous pemphigoid

↓

4. If none of the above, consider:
physical irritation
- heat, cold, radiation...

1.113.) <u>VAGINAL DISCHARGE</u>

	DISCHARGE	SYMPTOMS	WET SMEAR
Candida	thick curdy	pruritus	hyphae
Trichomonas	thin copious	discharge	motile protozoa
Gardnerella	scant non-irritating	odor [1]	"clue-cells" [2]

[1] fishy odor after 10% KOH ("whiff test")
[2] epithelial cells with attached bacteria

1.114.) <u>VERTIGO</u>

caloric test abnormal
(labyrinthine vertigo)

<u>AUDIOGRAM ABNORMAL</u>:
CT diagnostic
- acoustic neuroma
- glomus tumor

CT non-diagnostic
- ototoxic drugs
- Ménière's disease

<u>AUDIOGRAM NORMAL</u>:
- labyrinthitis
- chronic otitis media

spontaneous/optokinetic nystagmus
(central vertigo)

CT diagnostic
- multiple sclerosis
- meningioma
- intracranial aneurysms

CT non-diagnostic
- vertebrobasilar insufficiency
- migraine

VERTIGO	DIZZINESS
abnormal ENG	normal ENG
rotating sensation patient feels he is turning patient feels world is turning	fainting sensation
nausea, visual disturbances	

117

1.115.) <u>LOSS OF VISION - RETINAL</u>

	OPHTHALMOSCOPIC FINDINGS
retinal detachment	retinal bulge *patient describes veil over eye*
macular degeneration	**drusen** (discrete yellow deposits in macula) *central visual loss in elderly*
glaucoma ocular pressure > 20 mmHg	enlarged central cup *reduced visual field*
diabetic retinopathy	• "dot-n-blot" hemorrhages • hard or cotton wool exudates • microaneurysms • neovascularization
hypertensive retinopathy	• arteriolar narrowing • flame hemorrhages, exudates • arteriovenous nicking • "copper and silver wiring"
amaurosis fugax transient ischemic attacks	**cholesterol emboli** at arteriolar bifurcations (Hollenhorst plaques) *transient visual loss lasting seconds*
papilledema increased intracranial pressure mass lesions	blurred disc margins small cup absent venous pulse *minimal visual loss until late stage*

 WHO definition of blindness: vision < 1:20

1.116.) <u>VITAMIN B$_{12}$ DEFICIENCY</u>
(< 160 pg/mL)

1. Check methylmalonic acid and homocysteine levels
- to confirm borderline low cobalamin (100-200 pg/mL

2. If Schilling test (oral B12) is normal:
inadequate intake
- breast-fed infants
- alcoholics, strict vegetarians

increased requirements
- cancer
- hyperthyroidism

3. If Schilling test II (oral B12 plus IF) normal:
lack of intrinsic factor
- post gastrectomy
- gastric mucosal injury
- pernicious anemia

4. Schilling test III (oral B12 plus IF plus antibiotic) normal:
- bacterial overgrowth, "blind loop"

5. Schilling test III (oral B12 plus IF plus antibiotic) abnormal:
malabsorption
- sprue
- regional ileitis
- ileal resection

parasites
- fish tapeworm (*D. latum*)

drugs
- broad spectrum antibiotics

1.117.) WEIGHT GAIN

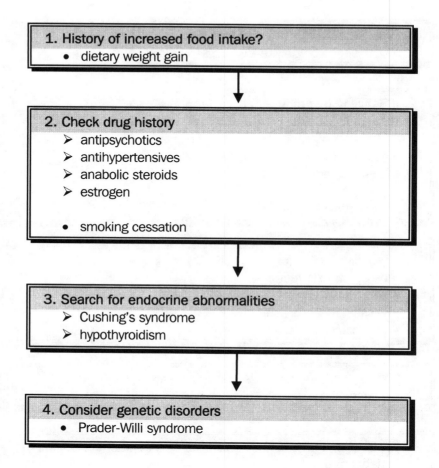

1. History of increased food intake?
- dietary weight gain

2. Check drug history
➢ antipsychotics
➢ antihypertensives
➢ anabolic steroids
➢ estrogen

- smoking cessation

3. Search for endocrine abnormalities
➢ Cushing's syndrome
➢ hypothyroidism

4. Consider genetic disorders
- Prader-Willi syndrome

1.118.) WEIGHT LOSS

1. Psychological evaluation
- stress, depression
- eating disorder

2. Consider HIV test in risk patients
- HIV

3. Rule out endocrine disorders
- diabetes mellitus
- hyperthyroidism
- Addison's disease

4. Get chest X-ray
- congestive heart failure
- COPD

4. Consider small bowel function tests
- inflammatory bowel disease
- sprue

5. Search for occult malignancies
- GI tract, liver
- leukemia, lymphoma

Hospital setting*: most likely serious disease*
Community setting*: likely stress/depression*

THERAPY
&
MANAGEMENT

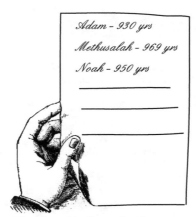

Adam – 930 yrs

Methusalah – 969 yrs

Noah – 950 yrs

_____

_____

The first Medicare bankruptcy

2.1.) <u>ABORTION (SPONTANEOUS)</u>

Risk factors	o age <15 years o age >35 years o chromosomal abnormalities o endometritis o cervical incompetence
Management	**1.** karyotype aborted fetus for genetic abnormalities **2.** consider cervical cerclage

 Vaginal bleeding in early pregnancy is common and usually does not present spontaneous abortion.

2.2.) <u>ABRUPTIO PLACENTAE</u>

Risk factors	o cocaine, smoking o multiparity o hypertension
Management	**1.** replace fluids and blood vigorously **2.** watch for signs of DIC
Prognosis	1% maternal mortality up to 50% fetal mortality

2.3.) <u>ACNE VULGARIS</u>

Risk factors	o male o androgens o anabolic steroids o oily cosmetics
Management	**1.** topical benzoyl peroxidase or tretinoin **2.** topical antibiotics **3.** oral antibiotics or isotretinoin

2.4.) <u>ACTINIC KERATOSIS</u>

Risk factors	o fair skin o high elevation o sun exposure
Management	**mild:** laser, cryo or other forms of dermabrasion **proliferative:** excision with margin
Prognosis	2-5% will progress to squamous cell carcinoma

2.5.) <u>ACUTE RENAL FAILURE</u>

Risk factors	
	o surgery
	o volume depletion
	➢ aminoglycosides
	➢ cyclosporine
	➢ ACE inhibitors
	➢ radio contrast

Prevention	
	• good hydration prior to contrast or chemotherapy
	• aggressive restoration of intravascular volume

1. Interstitial nephritis
- withdraw offending drug

↓

2. Acute tubular necrosis
- restore vascular fluid volume
- diuretics (but not if kidneys are obstructed!)

↓

3. Crescentic glomerulonephritis
- diagnosis needs to be made by renal biopsy
- steroids
- cyclophosphamide

2.6.) <u>ADDISON'S DISEASE</u>
(adrenal insufficiency)

Risk factors	o family history o prolonged intake of steroids o severe infection o severe trauma
2° Prevention	• prevent adrenal crisis • daily hydrocortisone • double dose during illness or preoperative
Management	**Acute:** hydrocortisone, IV replace Na and glucose **Chronic:** oral hydrocortisone patient should carry medic alert card

2.7.) <u>PRIMARY ALDOSTERONISM</u>

1. Adrenal adenoma
if unilateral:
• surgical removal → cure
if bilateral:
• aldosterone antagonist (spironolactone)
• ACE inhibitor

2. Bilateral zona glomerulosa hyperplasia
• aldosterone antagonist (spironolactone)
• ACE inhibitor

2.8.) <u>ALTITUDE SICKNESS</u>

Risk factors	o high altitude and rapid ascent o lack of conditioning
Prevention	• gradual ascent • good hydration ➢ acetazolamide
Management	**1.** descend!!! **2.** oxygen and/or hyperbaric bag **3.** dexamethasone to reduce cerebral edema **4.** nifedipine to reduce pulmonary distress
Complications	**pulmonary edema** → respiratory distress syndrome **cerebral edema** → seizures, coma, death

 Patients may resume ascent if symptoms resolve.

2.9.) <u>ALZHEIMER'S DISEASE</u>
most common cause of dementia

Risk factors	o age o positive family history o Down syndrome o aberrant apolipoprotein E
Management	➢ CNS cholinesterase inhibitor: donepezil ➢ antioxidants: vitamin E ➢ Gingko biloba

2.10.) AMYLOIDOSIS

Risk factors	**AL:** multiple myeloma other plasma cell disorders **AA:** chronic inflammatory diseases
Management	• control underlying chronic inflammation • renal involvement may require kidney transplant

2.11.) AMYOTROPHIC LATERAL SCLEROSIS

Risk factors	o age > 40 years o positive family history
Management	1. physical therapy to maintain patient's independence 2. provide psychological counseling 3. Baclofen for muscle cramps

2.12.) ANAPHYLACTIC SHOCK

Risk factors	o genetic predisposition o previous anaphylaxis
Prevention	• avoid drugs/food that cause reaction • wear medical ID • carry emergency epinephrine kit (insect stings)

1. If life-threatening:
- initial CPR, O_2, IV fluids
- epinephrine

↓

2. If not life-threatening, consider:
- epinephrine
- antihistamines
- glucocorticoids

↓

3. Monitor patient
- late reactions possible 6-12 hours after acute event
- consult with allergist

2.13.) ANKYLOSING SPONDYLITIS

Risk factors

- o male gender
- o Caucasians
- o HLA-B27
- o inflammatory bowel disease

Management

1. physical exercises are extremely important
2. maintain good posture
3. NSAIDs: indomethacin
4. if history of GI side effects: COX-2-selective NSAID

Other diseases associated with HLA-B27:
- o Reiter's Syndrome
- o uveitis
- o juvenile rheumatoid arthritis
- o psoriatic arthritis

2.14.) ANORECTAL ABSCESS

Risk factors

- o prolapsed hemorrhoids
- o inflammatory bowel disease
- o previous perirectal abscess

Prevention

- • avoid constipation
- • don't use enemas
- • perianal cleanliness

Management

- • incision and drainage
  (do not delay! do not "attempt" antibiotics!)

131

2.15.) ANOREXIA NERVOSA

Risk factors	o perfectionistic personality o high self-expectations o ambivalence about dependence/independence
Management	**1.** restore body weight / electrolytes (best done under hospital supervision) **2.** psychotherapy or family therapy
Prognosis	50% will achieve normal weight 6% will die → early onset indicates better prognosis

Rituals and abnormal attitudes towards food often persist.

2.16.) ANXIETY

Risk factors	o family history o lack of social support
prevention	• avoid stress • relaxation techniques • meditation
Management	• best results with antianxiety medication combined with long-term psychotherapy

2.17.) AORTIC DISSECTION

Risk factors	o hypertension o Marfan syndrome o Ehlers-Danlos syndrome o congenital aortic valve abnormalities o coarctation of aorta o trauma
Prognosis	10 year survival after surgery 60%

1. If it involves ascending aorta and arch:
- emergency surgery

2. If it involves descending aorta:
- medical management often sufficient
- surgery if distal ischemia develops

3. Follow-up
- good control of hypertension is most important
- CT or MRI to detect developing aneurysms

2.18.) AORTIC STENOSIS

Risk factors	**young adults:** congenital **adults:** rheumatic **elderly:** calcification
2° Prevention	• bacterial endocarditis prophylaxis • rheumatic fever prophylaxis • avoid exercise to prevent sudden death
Management	**1.** replace valve before left ventricular dysfunction occurs **2.** surgery is mandatory for symptomatic patients **3.** balloon dilatation is effective, but may lead to aortic insufficiency

Aortic stenosis is the second most fatal heart valve disease after mitral regurgitation

2.19.) APLASTIC ANEMIA

Risk factors	**hereditary** o Fanconi's anemia (autosomal recessive) **acquired** o viral illness o organic solvents o chloramphenicol
Management	**if HLA-identical sibling available:** • allogenic bone marrow transplant success rate is 60-70% **if no HLA-match is available:** • immunosuppression

2.20.) ARDS

(acute respiratory distress syndrome)

Any injury to alveolar epithelium can result in ARDS:

Risk factors	o toxic inhalation o sepsis o shock o diffuse pneumonia
Management	**1.** identify the cause **2.** mechanical ventilation **3.** try to avoid barotrauma to the lungs **4.** glucocorticoids for late phase ARDS (but not beneficial during acute stage)
Prognosis	50-70% mortality

 PEEP is used to increase oxygenation at a fixed P_{O_2}.

2.21.) ARTERIAL THROMBOSIS/EMBOLUS

Risk factors	**embolus**
	  o atrial flutter/fibrillation
	
	thrombosis
	  o atherosclerosis
	  o aneurysm
	  o vascular injury

Prevention	• anticoagulation • reduce risk factors for atherosclerosis
Management	1. anticoagulation with IV heparin 2. consider streptokinase to dissolve thrombus 3. if limb is in jeopardy → surgery

2.22.) ASPERGILLOSIS

Risk factors	**allergic:** exposure **aspergilloma:** pre-existing COPD, bronchiectasis, TB **systemic:** immunosuppression
Prevention	**allergic:** avoid dead plants, compost piles… **aspergilloma:** treat underlying lung disease
Management	1. itraconazole or amphotericin B for invasive aspergillosis 2. severe hemoptysis due to fungus ball may require surgery

2.23.) ASTHMA

Risk factors	o positive family history
2° Prevention	**avoid triggering factors:** • pollutants, dust, molds, cold, exercise **avoid aspirin**

---

1. Symptomatic relief:
- β-2 agonists: albuterol, terbutaline
- xanthines: theophylline

↓

2. Long-term control of disease:
- cromolyn (mast cell stabilizer)
- inhaled glucocorticoid
- inhaled glucocorticoid plus bronchodilator

↓

3. Status asthmaticus
- hospitalization
- monitor arterial blood gases
- oxygen
- IV glucocorticoids

Find the minimum level of treatment to suppress symptoms and teach patient to take responsibility for management of his disease.

2.24.) <u>ATELECTASIS (POSTOPERATIVE)</u>

Prevalence	• common in general anesthesia and ICU setting
Risk factors	o smoking o obesity
Prevention	• avoid 100% pure oxygen • early postoperative mobilization • aspiration precautions
Management	1. provide adequate pain control in surgical patients 2. chest physiotherapy: percussion, drainage 3. nasotracheal suction to remove secretions 4. antibiotics for pneumonia or bronchitis

2.25.) <u>ATOPIC DERMATITIS</u>

Risk factors	o genetic predisposition o emotional stress
3° Prevention	• avoid aggravating factors (cold, soaps, detergents, other irritants…)
Management	1. avoid drying of skin (soap, shampoos) 2. apply hydrophilic ointments (Eucerin) after bath or shower 3. tar shampoos reduce scalp itching 4. topical steroids (1% hydrocortisone) for inflamed areas

2.26.) <u>ATHEROSCLEROSIS</u>
leading cause of mortality/morbidity in Western countries

Risk factors	o hypertension o high LDL, low HDL o diabetes mellitus o smoking o obesity
Prevention	• reduce modifiable risk factors • **diet:** <30% of total calories from fat

2.27.) <u>ATRIAL FIBRILLATION</u>

Risk factors	o hypertension o rheumatic heart disease o left ventricular hypertrophy
Prevention	• long-term anticoagulation is required if atrial fibrillation recurs despite anti-arrhythmic therapy

Management	**acute fibrillations:** - calcium channel blockers
	           - beta blockers
	           - digoxin
	
	sustained fibrillations: attempt cardioversion [1]

[1] *patient MUST be anticoagulated beforehand (risk of embolus)!*

2.28.) ATRIAL SEPTAL DEFECT
10% of congenital heart defects

Risk factors	**ostium primum defect:** Down syndrome **ostium secundum defect:** most cases are sporadic
Management	**1.** Small defects may be left unrepaired. **2.** Surgical closure should be performed before pulmonary hypertension develops!
Complications	• atrial fibrillation • tricuspid regurgitation • right sided heart failure

2.29.) ADHD
Attention Deficit Hyperactivity Disorder

Risk factors	○ poor prenatal health
3° Prevention	• support and advice to lessen risk for abuse, depression, and social isolation
Management	**1.** assess parental involvement **2.** behavioral intervention **3.** consider Ritalin or dextroamphetamine (start at lowest dose, observe effect)

 Children with ADHD often develop antisocial personality disorder later in life.

140

2.30.) AUTISM

Risk factors	o male o genetic (high monozygotic twin concordance) o pregnancy complications o maternal rubella
Management	• lifelong need of supervised care (only 1-2% will become independent)

2.31.) AUTOIMMUNE HEMOLYTIC ANEMIA

Risk factors	**warm antibodies IgG (90%)** o "idiopathic" o leukemia, lymphoma, myeloma o drugs: methyldopa, quinidine…. **cold antibodies IgM (10%)** o "idiopathic" o mycoplasma, mononucleosis

Management	**1.** blood transfusion: monitor very carefully
	2. if renal impairment → aggressive hydration and
	                        diuresis
	3. search for underlying cause!
	
	warm antibodies: - glucocorticoids
	                       - consider splenectomy
	
	cold antibodies: - consider plasmapheresis

Most cases are "idiopathic".

2.32.) <u>BASAL CELL CARCINOMA</u>

Incidence	500,000 non-melanoma skin cancers/year in US (80% of these are BCC)
Risk factors	o sun exposure o fair skin
Prevention	• sunscreens, hat…
Prognosis	• metastatic potential 0.1%

Non-melanotic skin cancer is the most common cancer in the US, but usually excluded from cancer epidemiology tables because of its low fatality rate.

2.33.) <u>BENIGN PROSTATE HYPERPLASIA</u>

Risk factors	o increased estradiol levels with age
Management	**1.** digital rectal exam and PSA levels to rule out malignancy **2.** consider herbal remedies **3.** alpha blocker or 5α-reductase inhibitor **4.** TURP: transurethral resection of the prostate
Prognosis	Many patients will improve or stabilize even without treatment!

2.34.) BLADDER INJURY

Risk factors	o blunt trauma to lower abdomen o distended bladder at time of trauma o prior pelvic surgery
Prevention	• wear seat belts
Management	1. requires catheterization until hematuria resolves 2. rupture involving bladder neck → surgical repair 3. intraperitoneal ruptures → surgical repair

2.35.) BOTULISM

Risk factors	**food-borne:** home-canned food **infantile:** contaminated honey
Prevention	• no honey to infants <12 months of age
Management	1. support respiratory function 2. give *C. botulinum* antitoxin
Prognosis	10% mortality with intensive care

2.36.) <u>BRAIN ABSCESS</u>

Risk factors	o childhood poverty in developing countries o immunosuppression o IV drug abuse
Prevention	• early treatment of otitis media and dental abscesses • prophylactic antibiotics after penetrating head wounds
Management	1. be careful with lumbar puncture! 2. CSF → bacterial culture, antibiotic sensitivity 3. empirical antibiotic therapy (3rd Gen. Cephalosporin) 4. consider dexamethasone
Prognosis	10% mortality with early detection (CT or MRI) neurological sequelae in up to 50%

2.37.) <u>BREAST ABSCESS</u>

Risk factors	o puerperal mastitis o nipple retraction
Prevention	• early treatment of mastitis (milk expression, cold compresses, antibiotics)
Management	• nursing should be discontinued if abscess develops

2.38.) <u>BREAST CANCER</u>

Prevalence	1 in 8 women during lifetime
Risk factors	o positive family history o early menarche o late menopause o nulliparity o (high dietary fat)
2° Prevention	<u>Mammography</u> • baseline at 35 years • every 1-2 years between 40-50 years of age • every year after 50 years of age

1. Stage I (tumor < 2cm, no axillary nodes)
- lumpectomy with axillary lymph node resection
- *or* modified radical mastectomy
- ➤ consider adjuvant chemotherapy or hormonal therapy

↓

2. Stage II (tumor < 5cm or axillary node)
- same options as stage I
- plus radiation therapy if several lymph nodes are involved

↓

3. Stage III (tumor > 5cm or chest wall extension)
- preoperative chemotherapy
- followed by radical mastectomy

↓

4. Stage IV (metastatic)
- chemotherapy plus/minus hormonal therapy

2.39.) BREECH BIRTH

Risk factors	o low birth weight o prematurity o trisomy 21 o placenta previa
Management	• external version can be attempted at 30-36 weeks

2.40.) BRONCHIECTASIS

Caused by chronic, recurrent bacterial infections.

Risk factors	o foreign body aspiration o chronic respiratory infection
Prevention	• immunization pneumonia/influenza • treat pneumonia aggressively
Management	1. 2-4 weeks antibiotics (may have to try several different ones) 2. bronchodilators 3. percussion / postural drainage to clear secretions

 Less common nowadays thanks to antibiotics.

2.41.) BRONCHIOLITIS

Acute inflammation of small airways, usually caused by viruses.

Risk factors	newborns (2-6 months) children: day care environment
Prevention	• hand washing • avoid contact with infected persons
Management	1. correct hypoxemia if present 2. watch for dehydration due to tachypnea 3. consider ribavirin if due to RSV

2.42.) BRUCELLOSIS

Risk factors	o contact with cattle/sheep o unpasteurized milk o imported cheese
Prevention	• protective measures for meat and dairy workers • avoid fresh milk
Management	➤ Doxycycline

2.43.) <u>BURKITT'S LYMPHOMA</u>
(highly aggressive NHL)

Risk factors	90% of Burkitt's lymphoma in Africa a/w with EBV
Management	➤ high-dose chemotherapy regimen

2.44.) <u>BURNS</u>

1. Minor burns
- immediate cooling within 1st minute of burn decreases injury
- gentle débridement of loose tissue
- biologic dressing, sterile gauze
- apply topical antibiotic daily

↓

2. Major burns
- if > 10~20% of body surface area → refer to burn center
- if it involves face, hands or feet → refer to burn center

- replace fluids (Ringer's lactate)
- replace electrolytes (K, Ca, Mg, phosphate)
- replace albumin

- provide high caloric intake (if possible via GI tract)

Rule of 9:
Divide body surface area into 11 parts, each accounting for 9% of total:
Trunk = 4 · 9%,   each leg = 2 · 9%,   arms and head = 9% each.

148

2.45.) SYSTEMIC CANDIDIASIS

Risk factors	o immunosuppression o mucocutaneous candidiasis
Prevention	• antibiotic prophylaxis for chemotherapy or bone marrow transplant patients
Management	➢ fluconazole ➢ amphotericin B

2.46.) CONGENITAL CATARACT

Risk factors	o galactosemia o maternal diabetes o intrauterine infections (TORCH) [1] o glucocorticoids [1] o sulfonamides [1]
Management	**1.** surgical removal of lens material **2.** contact lenses

[1] *highest risk in first trimester*

 In 50-60% of cases no cause can be identified.

149

2.47.) CELIAC DISEASE

Risk factors	o family history o HLA-DR3
3° Prevention	• gluten-free diet (avoid wheat, barley, rye, oats)
Management	**1.** refer patient to dietitian **2.** replace vitamins and minerals **3.** 80% become symptom-free after several weeks/months on strict gluten-free diet

 Rice and corn are OK.

2.48.) CEREBRAL PALSY

Risk factors	o prematurity o hypoxia o perinatal seizures o meningitis/encephalitis
Management	**1.** physical therapy occupational therapy speech training **2.** should attend normal school if possible

2.49.) CERVICAL CANCER

Risk factors	**squamous carcinoma**
	   ○ human papilloma virus (types 16, 18, 31, 33…)
	   ○ smoking

Prevention	• monogamy
2° Prevention	• annual **Pap smear** for all sexually active women

---

1. Stage I (confined to cervix)
- modified radical hysterectomy
- if depth > 3mm → treatment like stage II

↓

2. Stage II (extends beyond cervix)
- radical hysterectomy or radiation therapy
  (equally effective, cure rate ~ 98%)
- if parametrium is affected → treat like stage III

↓

3. Stage III (extends to lower 1/3 of vagina)
4. Stage IV (extends beyond true pelvis)
- radiation therapy
- plus chemotherapy

 Do NOT combine surgery and radiation therapy!

2.50.) CHANCROID

Soft painful ulcers caused by *Haemophilus ducreyi*.

Risk factors	o multiple sexual partners o uncircumcised males o prostitute carriers
Prevention	• sexual counseling • condoms • treat partners
Management	➤ ceftriaxone or ciprofloxacin

2.51.) CHICKEN POX

Prevention	• active immunization for children > 1 years • passive immunization for immunocompromised
Management	• acetaminophen for fever • antipruritic creams or ointments ➤ acyclovir for immunocompromised patients
Complications	• pneumonia • encephalitis

 10% of adult population in US is susceptible.

2.52.) <u>CHLAMYDIA TRACHOMATIS</u>

most common STD in USA

Risk factors	o sexual promiscuity o lower socioeconomic groups
Prevention	• sexual counseling • screen "target population"
Management	➤ doxycycline
Complications	chronic PID is very common due to asymptomatic nature of the disease and non-compliance with treatment.

 Most women are asymptomatic for months or years!

153

2.53.) CHOLECYSTITIS

Prevalence	50% of patients with gallstones will develop symptoms
Risk factors	o cholelithiasis o biliary parasites

2.54.) CHOLELITHIASIS

Risk factors	o female o multiparity o obesity o rapid weight loss
Management	1. in most cases, removal of asymptomatic gallbladder is NOT recommended 2. attempt dissolution if asymptomatic (ursodeoxycholic acid)
Prognosis	1-2% of patients per year will develop symptoms requiring surgery

1. Acute cholecystitis
- broad-spectrum antibiotic
- place patient on NPO
- surgery after 24-48 hours

2. Chronic cholecystitis
- elective laparoscopic cholecystectomy

2.55.) CHOLERA

Risk factors	o travel to epidemic areas o contaminated food, water
Prevention	• water purification • no unpeeled raw fruits/vegetables • tetracycline for contacts • prophylactic vaccine is NOT recommended
Management	1. if comatose → Ringer's lactate 2. ORS: Oral Rehydration Solution (WHO formula) to replace fluid and electrolytes lost with stool 3. tetracycline/doxycycline
Prognosis	mortality <1% if treated with ORS

2.56.) CLUSTER HEADACHE

Risk factors	o male o age > 30 years o vasodilators
Prophylaxis	• ergotamine at bedtime • avoid nitroglycerin and vasodilator drugs • avoid alcohol
Management	1. O_2 by mask often effective 2. try methysergide, glucocorticoid or sumatriptan 3. if intractable → trigeminal blockade

155

2.57.) <u>CMV INFECTION</u>

50-100% of population is seropositive

Risk factors	o organ transplantation o immunosuppression o AIDS
Prevention	• if patient is seronegative for CMV, try to avoid transplanting organ from CMV positive donor
Management	➤ ganciclovir for disseminated infection
Prognosis	major cause of morbidity in organ transplant patients (especially bone marrow transplants) CMV pneumonia in these patients >80% mortality

 Risk of intrauterine infection 50-100% with primary maternal infection during pregnancy.

2.58.) <u>COARCTATION OF AORTA</u>

Risk factors	o other congenital heart abnormalities o Turner's syndrome
Management	• resection of narrowed segment (10-year survival after surgery >90%)

156

2.59.) <u>COCCIDIOIDOMYCOSIS</u>

Risk factors	○ endemic to Southwest of US ○ lab cultures are highly contagious! ○ high risk of disseminated disease in AIDS patients
Prevention	• avoid exposure (especially high risk population)
Management	**1.** if uncomplicated → observe **2.** if pulmonary or disseminated disease → itraconazole

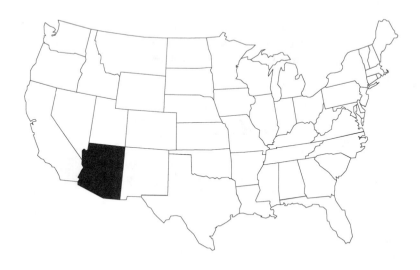

2.60.) <u>COLORECTAL CANCER</u>

Risk factors

- o ulcerative colitis
- o familial polyposis
- o adenomatous polyps

- o high dietary animal fat
- o low dietary fiber intake

Management

<u>COLON CANCER</u>
1. surgical resection
2. resection plus chemotherapy for Duke C
3. postoperative screening: CEA, endoscopy or CT yearly

<u>RECTAL CANCER</u>
1. preoperative radiotherapy

Prognosis

		<u>5-year survival</u>
Duke A	(mucosa and submucosa)	- 95%
Duke B1	(muscularis)	- 85%
Duke B2	(through serosa)	- 75%
Duke C	(regional lymph nodes)	- 45%
Duke D	(distant metastases)	- 5%

2.61.) <u>CONSTIPATION</u>

Risk factors

- o sedentary lifestyle
- o drugs: anticholinergics

Management

1. high fiber diet (20-30g fiber/day)
2. increase fluid intake
3. bowel training

2.62.) <u>CONTACT DERMATITIS</u>

Risk factors	o cosmetics o jewelry o occupational exposure
Management	**1.** avoid exposure **2.** use gloves with cotton lining

2.63.) <u>COPD</u>

Risk factors	o smoking o passive smoking, air pollution o viral pneumonia in early life o airway hyperreactivity o α1-antitrypsin deficiency
Prevention	• stop smoking • immunize against pneumonia and influenza
Management	**1.** symptomatic relief - bronchodilators - glucocorticoids for acute inflammation - broad-spectrum antibiotics **2.** proper nutrition is important **3.** late stage → consider lung volume reduction surgery **4.** monitor lung function (FEV_1) **5.** annual chest X-ray

 COPD with predominant bronchitis has better prognosis than with predominant emphysema.

2.64.) CORONARY ARTERY DISEASE

causes 1/3 of deaths in US (myocardial infarction)

Risk factors

- o male gender
- o hypertension
- o smoking
- o high LDL
- o low HDL
- o obesity
- o diabetes mellitus

Management

1. recommend low fat/low cholesterol diet
2. promote smoking cessation
3. control blood pressure
4. consider prophylactic aspirin
5. estrogen replacement in postmenopausal women

Prognosis

<u>risk of myocardial infarction</u>
- the relative risk of smokers approaches that of non-smokers within 2-3 years of smoking cessation

- 1% decrease in serum cholesterol lowers risk by 2-3%
- 1 mmHG decrease in blood pressure lowers risk 2-3%
- maintaining active lifestyle lowers risk 45%

Treadmill stress test is NOT recommended as routine screening in adults with no evidence of coronary heart disease.

Dietary goals to prevent heart disease:
less than 2 risk factors: LDL <160 mg/dL
2 or more risk factors: LDL <130 mg/dL
coronary heart disease: LDL <100 mg/dL

2.65.) COR PULMONALE

Risk factors	o living at high altitude
	o smoking
Prevention	• stop smoking
Prognosis	COPD with cor pulmonale: 50% mortality in 3 years

2.66.) CROHN'S DISEASE

Risk factors	o Caucasians
	o Jewish ancestry
	o family history
	o major psychological stress → trigger
Prognosis	- worse than ulcerative colitis
	- mortality increases with duration of disease

---

1. Mild to moderate disease
- sulfasalazine (more effective for colon than small bowels)
- antibiotics

2. Severe disease
- glucocorticoids for acute phase
  (should be tapered as soon as remission occurs)
- mercaptopurine or azathioprine to sustain remission
- experimental: antibodies to tumor necrosis factor!
- unresponsive, or obstructions → surgery

2.67.) CRYPTOCOCCOSIS

Risk factors	o immunosuppression - reactivation of latent lung foci → pneumonia - dissemination, meningitis
Prevention	• avoid pigeon droppings • itraconazole prophylaxis for AIDS patients
Management	➢ itraconazole

2.68.) CRYPTORCHIDISM

Risk factors	o prematurity o family history
Management	**1.** try hCG to promote testicular descent **2.** surgery (orchiopexy) at age of 1 year **3.** orchiectomy if discovered post puberty
Prognosis	- decreased fertility rate - 10-50 fold risk of seminoma

Orchiopexy does NOT reduce risk of malignant degeneration but facilitates early detection.

2.69.) CUSHING'S SYNDROME

Causes	**most common cause:** iatrogenic **other causes:** 80% pituitary 20% adrenal
Risk factors	• prolonged use of glucocorticoids
Management	1. transphenoidal removal of pituitary adenoma 2. if this fails, consider bilateral adrenalectomy 3. lifelong mineralocorticoid and glucocorticoid replacement after total adrenalectomy

2.70.) CUTANEOUS DRUG REACTIONS

Risk factors	○ penicillin, sulfonamides, many more…
Prevention	**beware of potential crossover reactions:** penicillin ↔ cephalosporins hydantoin ↔ carbamazepine ↔ barbiturates
Management	1. topical antipruritics 2. antihistamines 3. systemic glucocorticoids for severe cases

2.71.) CYSTIC FIBROSIS

most common lethal genetic disease in Caucasians

Risk factors	o family history o Ashkenazi Jews
Management	**1.** daily chest physical therapy (percussion) **2.** annual influenza immunization **3.** avoid general anesthesia
Prognosis	average life expectancy now ~30 years

2.72.) DEEP VEIN THROMBOSIS

Risk factors	o prolonged immobility o pregnancy o oral contraceptives o malignancies
Prevention	• low-dose heparin • low-dose warfarin • compression stockings • low estrogen content birth control pills
Management	**1.** initial anticoagulation with heparin (monitor APTT) **2.** oral anticoagulation with warfarin (monitor INR: 2~3) (for 3-6 months) **3.** if anticoagulation is contraindicated: vena cava filter
Prognosis	20% of untreated DVT develop pulmonary emboli (of these ~10% are fatal)

2.73.) <u>DEMENTIA</u>

Risk factors	o age o family history o atherosclerosis o head trauma, CNS infection
Management	**1.** *Gingko biloba* may improve memory **2.** safety first: avoid alcohol, driving, etc. **3.** wear medic alert card
Prognosis	**Alzheimer-type:** always progressive **Multi-infarct type:** not always progressive

2.74.) <u>DIABETES MELLITUS - TYPE 1</u>
(IDDM)

Risk factors	o HLA-DR3 o HLA-DR4 o monozygotic twin concordance 30%

1. Insulin
- morning dose before breakfast
- evening dose before dinner
- mix intermediate (NPH) with short acting (regular) insulins

2. Family education is most important!
- carbohydrate counting, regular meal times
- physical exercise: reduce insulin or provide extra snack

3. Follow-up
- quarterly physical exam, including HBA_{1c}

2.75.) <u>DIABETES MELLITUS TYPE 2</u>
(NIDDM)

Prevalence	2% of population
Risk factors	o gestational diabetes o monozygotic twin concordance 100%
Prevention	• avoid obesity • exercise
Management	**1.** sulfonylureas (short acting are more safe) **2.** metformin decreases hepatic gluconeogenesis **3.** insulin often required for endstage type II

 >10% of US population has impaired glucose tolerance, but only some progress to overt diabetes mellitus.

2.76.) <u>DIABETIC HYPOGLYCEMIA</u>

Prevalence	more common in type 1
Risk factors	o gastroenteritis o more common in "tightly controlled" patients treated for several years
Prevention	• patient education • routine schedule/diet
Management	**1.** oral glucose (fruit juice) **2.** if unable to take oral → glucagon **3.** if comatose → IV glucose

166

2.77.) <u>DIABETIC KETOACIDOSIS</u>

Prevalence	more common in type 1
Risk factors	o physical/emotional stress o trauma o infections o vomiting
Prevention	• monitor glucose during stressful situations
Management	1. fluid replacement (0.9% saline) 2. insulin infusion (monitor glucose) 3. monitor K^+ hourly → add to infusion when it starts to drop due to redistribution 4. bicarbonate for severe acidosis (pH<7)

Hyperosmolar coma is more common than diabetic ketoacidosis in adults and elderly with type 2 diabetes.

2.78.) <u>DIABETIC RETINOPATHY</u>
major cause of blindness in US

Risk factors	o duration of diabetes mellitus o poor glucose control o systemic hypertension
Prevention	• tight control of blood glucose (monitor HbA_{1c}) • aggressive treatment of hypertension

2.79.) DIPHTHERIA

Risk factors	o inadequate immunization o minority racial groups
Prevention	**Immunization:** • DPT at 2,4,6 and 15 months • booster every 10 years

Management	**1.** hospitalize (ICU)
	2. give antitoxin
	   - don't wait for bacterial culture!
	   - monitor closely for hypersensitivity reaction!
	3. penicillin

2.80.) DISCOID LUPUS ERYTHEMATOSUS

Risk factors	o female o African American o systemic lupus erythematosus
Management	**1.** avoid sun exposure **2.** avoid excessive heat or cold **3.** avoid skin trauma

2.81.) <u>DISSOCIATIVE DISORDERS</u>

(1.) Dissociative amnesia: memory gaps from minutes to days.
(2.) Fugue: patient assumes new name, identity and behavior but may appear normal
(3.) Identity disorder: multiple personalities alternate and "take over" patient's behavior.
(4.) Depersonalization disorder: feeling of being detached from self

Risk factors	o neglect, abuse, trauma during childhood
Prevention	• child abuse prevention • crisis intervention
Management	• supportive, stable environment • psychotherapy - consider hypnosis for identity disorder • consider antianxiety medication

2.82.) <u>DIVERTICULOSIS</u>

Prevalence	20-50% of US population over 50 years
Risk factors	o age o low fiber diet
Management	**DIVERTULOSIS** • high fiber diet (20-30g/day) • bulk forming laxatives (psyllium, methylcellulose) • if bleeding → sigmoidoscopy, angiography **DIVERTICULITIS** • antibiotics, bowel rest • signs of peritonitis → hospitalize, IV antibiotics • may require surgery

2.83.) DROWNING

Risk factors	o alcohol o inadequate supervision of children
Management	**1.** hypothermia slows metabolism → always attempt resuscitation, even if patient was submerged long time **2.** don't waste time trying to remove water from lungs **3.** begin mouth-mouth and cardiac compression **4.** if diving accident: suspect neck injury and stabilize **5.** hospitalize, even if patient seems to recover!

```
MOST COMMON CAUSES OF ACCIDENTS:
#1 - motor vehicle accidents
#2 - falls
#3 - poisoning
#4 - burns
#5 - drowning
```

2.84.) DYSMENORRHEA

Prevalence	40% of adult females have menstrual pain 10% are incapacitated for a few days each month
Risk factors	**primary dysmenorrhea** o nulliparity **secondary dysmenorrhea** o endometriosis o pelvic infection o STDs
Prevention	• reduce risk of STDs
Management	**1.** NSAIDs: ibuprofen **2.** daily calcium supplement **3.** oral contraceptives **4.** antidepressant (fluoxetine) during luteal phase

170

2.85.) <u>DYSPAREUNIA</u>

Prevalence	1-2% of adult females
Risk factors	o endometriosis o diabetes mellitus o estrogen deficiency o menopause
Management	**1.** examine both partners **2.** provide counseling in sex techniques **3.** lidocaine cream

2.86.) <u>DYSPEPSIA</u>

Risk factors	o other functional disorders o anxiety o depression
Management	**1.** frequent small meals **2.** avoid: 　- coffee and tea 　- chocolate 　- alcohol and smoking 　- NSAIDs **3.** search for underlying cause: 　- esophageal reflux 　- ulcer disease 　- *H. pylori* infection

2.87.) ECLAMPSIA

Risk factors	o primigravida o twin gestation o hydatidiform mole o preexisting renal disease or hypertension
HELLP	hepatic injury due to preeclampsia: • Hemolysis • Elevated Liver enzymes • Low Platelets
Prognosis	• most cases of preeclampsia are mild • severe preeclampsia often due to preexisting renal disease or autoimmune disorders

---

1. Preeclampsia
- good prenatal care improves outcome
- control of preexisting hypertension
- bed rest
- magnesium sulfate

2. Eclampsia
- place patient in lateral position
- magnesium sulfate IV for convulsions
- monitor fetal viability
- when mother is stabilized → delivery

Hypertension developing during pregnancy increases the likelihood of later "essential" hypertension.

2.88.) ECTOPIC PREGNANCY

(most common cause of maternal death in first half of pregnancy in US)

Risk factors	o pelvic inflammatory disease o use of IUD o endometritis o "morning after pill"
Prevention	• ultrasound to verify location of pregnancy to prevent complications of ectopic pregnancy (tubal rupture)
Management	**1.** if early → methotrexate (DNA synthesis inhibitor) **2.** if late → laparoscopic surgery **3.** follow-up: hCG levels

173

2.89.) <u>ENCEPHALITIS - VIRAL</u>

Risk factors	**Winter:** Mumps, Varicella **Summer:** Arthropod-borne viruses **Summer/Fall:** Enteroviruses
Management	**1.** examine CSF for diagnosis **2.** consider PCR of CSF to detect viral DNA or RNA **3.** acyclovir for herpes encephalitis foscarnet: wide-spectrum anti-viral
Prognosis	neurologic sequelae in 10-80% depending on virus **worst prognosis:** EEE and herpes simplex[1]

[1] *Herpes encephalitis is treatable! Early diagnosis is crucial!*

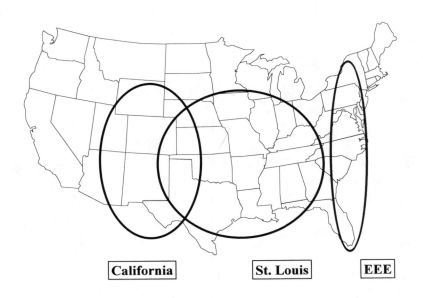

| California | St. Louis | EEE |

174

2.90.) <u>ENDOCARDITIS (bacterial)</u>

Risk factors	o IV catheters o IV drug abuse o artificial valves o acquired valve dysfunction
Prevention	• maintain good oral hygiene • antibiotic prophylaxis prior to dental procedures
Management	**1.** empirical antibiotics: nafcillin + gentamicin (don't wait for result of culture!) **2.** vancomycin for penicillin-resistant staphylococci

2.91.) <u>ENDOMETRIAL CARCINOMA</u>
most common gynecologic malignancy

Risk factors	o age >40 years o early menarche o late menopause o nulliparity o obesity
Prevention	• avoid unopposed estrogen

---

1. Stage I (limited to endometrium)
2. Stage II (extends to cervix)
• hysterectomy and bilateral salpingo-oophorectomy

3. Stage III (confined to true pelvis)
4. Stage IV (invading bladder/rectum)
• as above, plus add radiotherapy or chemotherapy
• consider hormonal therapy (progesterone)

2.92.) ENDOMETRIOSIS

Prevalence	10% of women of reproductive age
Prevention	• pregnancy may have positive effect

Management	1. hormone therapy
	   - oral contraceptives
	   - progesterone only to induce amenorrhea
	   - danazol (steroid receptor blocker) to induce amenorrhea
	2. surgery
	   - laparoscopic removal of lesions

2.93.) ENURESIS

Prevalence	10% of children
Risk factors	o male o first born child o family history

Management	1. wetting alarms
	2. drugs:
	   - imipramine
	   - anticholinergics

2.94.) EPIGLOTTITIS

Prevalence	dramatically decreased since *H. influenza* vaccine
Risk factors	o children 2-4 years
Management	1. Rifampin for household and day care contacts 2. intubation may be necessary for 24-48 hours

 This is a medical emergency!

2.95.) EPILEPSY

1. Pharmacotherapy
- "start low, go slow"
- may have to try several drugs
- after 2 seizure-free years, drugs may be withdrawn
  careful: → taper off slowly

- ➤ **partial seizures:** try carbamazepine
- ➤ **generalized seizures:** try valproic acid

↓

2. Pregnancy
- usually, the risk of discontinuing medication is larger than the risk of fetal abnormalities due to drug.

↓

3. Status epilepticus
- keep airways open
- lorazepam IV
- if seizures do not stop may require general anesthesia

2.96.) ERYSIPELAS

Risk factors	o skin lesions, abrasions o stasis dermatitis o diabetes o immunosuppression
Management	• penicillin • if recurrent, search for source of streptococcal infection

2.97.) ERYTHEMA INFECTIOSUM
(fifth disease, human parvovirus B19)

Prevention	• standard hygiene practices • contagious period is before rash appears
Management	• symptomatic treatment of headache and fever
Complications	• risk of intrauterine infection • risk of aplastic crisis in sickle cell patients

 Pregnant women should avoid patients with aplastic crisis.

2.98.) ERYTHROBLASTOSIS FETALIS

Prevalence	most cases now due to ABO incompatibility most severe cases still due to Rh incompatibility
Risk factors	o Rh-positive fetus in Rh-negative woman o prior transfusion of incompatible blood *Risk of sensitization without prophylaxis about 10%.*
Prevention	1. RhoGAM at 28-32 weeks for unsensitized women (negative indirect Coombs test) 2. postpartum RhoGAM if baby is Rh-positive

1. Maternal management
- monitor Rh antibody titers in Rh negative women
- if sensitized, perform amniocentesis → bilirubin

2. Fetal management
- consider intravascular blood transfusion
  (into umbilical vein)
- glucocorticoids to accelerate fetal lung maturation
- deliver early (28 weeks)

3. Neonatal management
- assess hematocrit and bilirubin levels
- phototherapy to avoid kernicterus

2.99.) ESOPHAGEAL CANCER

Risk factors	squamous cell carcinoma (most common worldwide)
	  o smoking
	  o alcohol
	
	adenocarcinoma (most common in US)
	  o Barrett's metaplasia

Prevention	• stop smoking • limit alcohol
Management	1. if early and limited to mucosa → surgical resection 2. if advanced (most patients) → chemotherapy or radiation followed by surgery
Prognosis	5-year survival 5-10%

2.100.) FALLOT'S TETRALOGY

(1.) ventricular septal defect
(2.) overriding aorta
(3.) pulmonary stenosis
(4.) → right ventricular hypertrophy

Prevalence	most common cyanotic heart disease after age 1y.
Management	• fatal unless surgically corrected

180

2.101.) FEBRILE SEIZURES

Prevalence	3-5% of children have one febrile seizure before age 5y.
Management	**1.** acetaminophen prophylaxis during fever **2.** diazepam prophylaxis <u>during high fever</u> continuous prophylaxis is controversial
Prognosis	• 70% one episode only • most recurrences within 1 year • risk of later epilepsy 2-3%

2.102.) FIBROCYSTIC CHANGE

 This is NOT a disease. The term "Fibrocystic breast disease" should be avoided.

Prevalence	>50% of adult women
Prevention	avoiding caffeine may reduce breast pain
Prognosis	no increase in cancer risk

<u>RELATIVE RISK FOR BREAST CANCER:</u>

no increased cancer risk:	fibrosis fibroadenoma mastitis squamous metaplasia
1.5-2fold cancer risk:	florid adenosis hyperplasia
5fold cancer risk:	atypical hyperplasia

2.103.) FOOD ALLERGY

Prevalence	1-2% of adults, more common in children
Risk factors	o atopic predisposition
Management	• avoid offending food
Prognosis	**infants:** usually outgrow their hypersensitivity **adults:** allergy often persists

*"Perceived" food allergy is much more common than "true"
food allergy.*

2.104.) FRAGILE-X SYNDROME

second most common genetic cause of mental retardation (after Down syndrome)

Risk factors	o fragile site on long arm of chromosome X
Prevention	• genetic counseling (X-linked recessive disorder) • consider amniocentesis
Prognosis	**males:** mild to moderate retardation **females:** lower expression of disease than males

2.105.) GANGRENE

Risk factors	o arteriosclerosis o diabetes mellitus o smoking o trauma
Prevention	• good skin care • avoid trauma
Management	**1.** reduce risk factors for atherosclerosis! **2.** regular exercise for patients with claudication **3.** get surgical consultation → revascularization

2.106.) GASTRIC ADENOCARCINOMA

Incidence	dramatic decrease in US for unknown reasons
Risk factors	o pickled, salted, spicy Asian food o food nitrates o smoking o polyposis
2° Prevention	• Endoscopic screening in endemic areas (Japan)

Management	**1.** early disease
	  - resection
	  - adjuvant chemotherapy is investigational
	2. late disease
	  - chemotherapy
	  - surgery of palliative value only

Gastric Lymphoma (MALT) has been linked to H. pylori and has a much better prognosis than adenocarcinoma.

2.107.) CHRONIC GASTRITIS TYPE A
(affects mostly corpus)

Prevalence	much less common than type B chronic gastritis
Risk factors	o antibodies to parietal cells o antibodies to intrinsic factor
Management	• lifelong parenteral Vit. B12 prevents pernicious anemia

2.108.) CHRONIC GASTRITIS TYPE B
(affects mostly antrum)

Prevalence	up to 80% of population >50 years
Risk factors	o *H. pylori* infection
Management	**TRIPLE THERAPY** 1. proton pump inhibitor (omeprazole) 2. plus amoxicillin 3. plus tetracycline or metronidazole
Prognosis	• increased risk of gastric cancer • increased risk of lymphoma (MALT)

2.109.) <u>EROSIVE GASTRITIS</u>

Risk factors	
	o shock
	o burns
	o sepsis
	o trauma
Management	**ICU patients:** antacids or H$_2$-blockers
	NSAID users: misoprostol

Overt bleeding from erosive gastritis in an ICU setting has very high mortality!

2.110.) <u>GASTROESOPHAGEAL REFLUX DISEASE</u>

Risk factors	
	foods that lower LES pressure:
	o chocolate, mint
	irritant foods:
	o lemon juice, spicy tomato juice
	other:
	o smoking, alcohol, coffee
Management	**1.** diet modification
	2. antacids: histamine (H2) antagonists
	3. annual endoscopy in patients with Barrett's metaplasia

2.111.) GIARDIASIS

most common cause of water-borne gastroenteritis in US

Risk factors	<ul><li>camping</li><li>day care centers</li><li>male homosexuality</li></ul>
Prevention	<ul><li>hand washing</li><li>water purification/boiling when camping</li></ul>
Management	➤ metronidazole

2.112.) GLAUCOMA

Prevalence	90% of these are chronic, open angle
Risk factors	<ul><li>family history</li><li>African Americans</li></ul>

Acute angle-closure glaucoma (=medical emergency!)

1. Induce miosis
- pilocarpine, carbachol

2. Reduce aqueous production
- topical β-blocker
- carbonic anhydrase inhibitor

3. Laser iridotomy of <u>both</u> eyes

↓

2. Chronic open-angle glaucoma
- control intraocular pressure (IOP), medical or laser
- regular assessment of IOP and visual fields

2.113.) POSTSTREPTOCOCCAL GLOMERULONEPHRITIS

Prevalence	leading cause of acute nephritic syndrome
Risk factors	o streptococcal infection in children 2-6 years (~15% risk after infection with nephritogenic strain)
Prevention	• treat streptococcal infections aggressively
Management	1. antihypertensives 2. salt restriction 3. diuretics (glucocorticoids are not useful)

2.114.) GONORRHEA

Risk factors	o multiple sexual partners
Prevention	• condoms • identify and treat sexual partners
Management	➤ single dose ceftriaxone plus 7-days doxycycline

2.115.) <u>GOUT</u>

Prevalence	**hyperuricemia:** 2-10% of population **gout:** 5% of patients with hyperuricemia
Risk factors	o obesity o diuretics o rapid cell turnover

---

1. Acute Gout
- avoid aspirin!
- NSAIDs: indomethacin
- oral colchicine (inhibits neutrophils)
- oral or intra-articular glucocorticoids

2. Chronic gout
- reduce risk factors
- allopurinol (inhibits uric aid synthesis)
- consider low-dose colchicine prophylaxis

Lifelong suppression of uric acid may be necessary if attacks recur.

2.116.) <u>GUILLAIN-BARRÉ SYNDROME</u>

Risk factors	o viral infection 1-3 weeks earlier
Management	1. confirm diagnosis with CSF 2. constant monitoring and support of vital functions 3. immune globulin infusion 4. plasmapheresis
Prognosis	• mortality 3% • 30% require ventilatory assistance • 10% have severe neurological residua

2.117.) <u>HEATSTROKE</u>

Risk factors	o elderly, bedridden patients o use of anticholinergics, diuretics o salt and water deprivation o alcohol o obesity
Management	1. rapid cooling (ice water bath) 2. IV fluids and electrolytes

Most patients recover within 30 minutes of collapse.

2.118.) HEMOCHROMATOSIS

Risk factors	o male [1] o alcohol (increases iron absorption)
2° Prevention	• screen family members !
Management	1. weekly phlebotomy to remove excess iron (less frequent after iron stores normalize) 2. deferoxamine - iron chelation

[1] *Clinical expression of disease is 10fold lower in women compared to men (due to protective effect of monthly menstruation)*

2.119.) HEMOPHILIA

Prevalence	hemophilia A is 10x more common than B
2° Prevention	• genetic counseling

---

1. Factor VIII and IX concentrates
- nowadays virus-inactivated and safe from HIV
- small risk of hepatitis C remains
- recombinant factor products are safest

↓

2. Other agents
- DDAVP (vasopressin analogue, available as nasal spray) increases factor VIII levels by unknown mechanism

---

10-20% of patients with hemophilia A will develop inhibitors (IgG) against factor VIII.

2.120.) HEPATITIS

Prevalence (positive serology)	**HAV:** 20-40% (up to 100% in developing countries) **HBV:** 5-10% **HCV:** 1-2%
Risk factors	**HAV:** fecal-oral route, poor sanitation **HBV:** body fluids, perinatal, male homosexuality **HCV:** IV-drug abuse, blood transfusions
Prevention	**HAV:** good sanitation **HBV:** screen all pregnant women vaccinate infants at birth
Management	**1.** no special treatment required in most cases **2.** bed rest or dietary restrictions are unnecessary **3.** chronic active viral hepatitis: consider interferon-α and ribavirin
Prognosis	**HBV:** 4% chronic active hepatitis → cirrhosis 5-10% asymptomatic HBsAg carrier (up to 100% carrier rate if neonatal infection) **HCV:** 50% chronic active hepatitis → cirrhosis

90% of transfusion-related hepatitis due to HCV. Becomes rarer with second-generation anti-HCV screening of blood products.

2.121.) <u>HEPATOCELLULAR ADENOMA</u>

Prevalence	- exceedingly rare prior to oral-contraceptive era - occur almost all in females
Risk factors	o estrogen
Management	**1.** discontinue oral contraceptives **2.** avoid pregnancy (risk of rupture and bleeding) **3.** if large → surgical removal

2.122.) <u>HEPATOCELLULAR CARCINOMA</u>

Risk factors	o males o liver cirrhosis (80% of cases) o HBV o HCV o aflatoxin
Prevention	• HBV and HCV prevention • consider AFP screening in high risk population
Prognosis	- radio- and chemotherapy usually unsuccessful - liver transplantation limited by recurrence, metastases

2.123.) HEPATORENAL SYNDROME
(renal failure in liver disease)

Risk factors	o reduction in effective blood volume
Prevention	• avoid vigorous abdominal paracentesis • avoid excessive diuresis • albumin replacement
Prognosis	no effective therapy, almost always fatal

2.124.) HERPES SIMPLEX INFECTION

Prevalence	**HSV I:** 80-90% of population seropositive **HSV II:** 20% of population seropositive
Risk factors	o unprotected sexual intercourse o immune compromise (stress, illness) o neonates (via birth canal)
Management	**1.** avoid sexual contact while disease active **2.** C. section if genital herpetic lesions present **3.** acyclovir for serious or systemic disease

30% transmission rate if vaginal delivery during primary episode of mother.

HSV-II is an independent risk factor for transmission of HIV.

2.125.) HERPES ZOSTER
(shingles)

Risk factors	o age o immunocompromise
Management	1. wet compresses to relief itching 2. analgesics 3. acyclovir for immunocompromised patients

 Zoster patients may transmit Varicella virus to susceptible persons → chicken pox.

2.126.) HIP FRACTURE
= fracture of proximal femur

Risk factors	o osteoporosis
Prevention	• osteoporosis prophylaxis • walking cane
Management	• internal fixation • consider hip arthroplasty for femur neck fractures • rapid mobilization is important!

2.127.) <u>HISTOPLASMOSIS</u>

Risk factors	**bird droppings:** o excavation o bull dozing o cave exploration
Management	**1.** acute pulmonary disease: none required **2.** chronic or disseminated disease : itraconazole **3.** lifelong itraconazole maintenance for AIDS patients
Prognosis	**pulmonary histoplasmosis:** resolves spontaneously **AIDS patients:** up to 50% relapse despite therapy

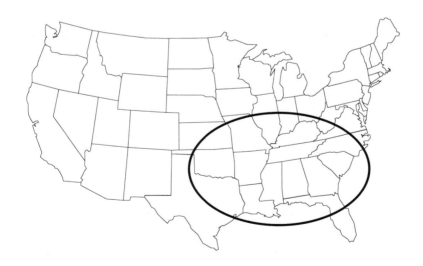

2.128.) HIV INFECTION

Prevalence	more than 700,000 reported cases in US since beginning of epidemic

Risk factors	**1. sexual contact**
	  o homosexual
	  o heterosexual
	
	2. percutaneous injury
	    (needle stick)
	
	3. mucous membranes exposed to contaminated blood
	
	4. mother to infant (vertical transmission)
	  o prenatal
	  o perinatal
	
	5. breast feeding

Prevention	• practice safe sex • sexual counseling for teenagers • needle exchange programs
Prognosis	life expectancy has improved due to new drug regimens

 Risk of HIV infection after needle stick injury is about 1:250

> ➢ Risk of HIV infection to fetus of HIV positive mother 10-40%.
> ➢ This can be reduced by 70% if AZT is given to the mother during pregnancy.

1. Initial evaluation
- HIV serology
- CD4 count
- asses presence of hepatitis, CMV, toxoplasma
- tuberculin test

- offer Pneumovax
- offer Hepatitis A and B vaccination

2. Monitor development of disease
- CD4 count every 3-6 months
- or check viral RNA load

3. Antiretroviral therapy
- **start if CD4 < 500 or HIV RNA > 20,000**

reverse transcriptase inhibitors (nucleosides)
- zidovudine (AZT)
- didanosine (ddI)

reverse transcriptase inhibitors (non-nucleosides)
- nevirapine (NVP)

protease inhibitors
- saquinavir (SQV

2. If CD4 <200
- trimethoprim-sulfamethoxazole prophylaxis for PCP

Always use combination therapy to prevent development of resistance. Initial therapy for example could be 2 or 3 nucleoside analogues plus a protease inhibitor.

2.129.) HODGKIN'S DISEASE

Incidence	bimodal distribution: young adults + elderly
Risk factors	o male o immunodeficiency o (EBV infection in some cases)

B symptoms: weight loss, fever, night sweats

---

1. Stage I (single lymph node region)
2. Stage II (several lymph node regions on same side of diaphragm)
- if no B symptoms: radiate affected lymph node regions
- if B symptoms: chemotherapy plus/minus radiation

---

3. Stage III (several lymph node regions on both sides of diaphragm)
4. Stage IV (involves extranodal sites)
- 6 to 8 cycles of chemotherapy:

MOPP: mechlorethamine + vincristine + procarbazine + prednisone
ABVD: doxorubicin + bleomycin + vinblastine + dacarbazine

---

5. Relapse
- consider high-dose chemotherapy with autologous stem cell transplant

Patients with splenectomy require Pneumovax vaccine.

2.130.) HUNTINGTON'S CHOREA

Risk factors	o family history
Management	• genetic counseling: ½ of offspring is potentially affected (offer DNA test to family members)
Prognosis	• fatal within 20 years • early onset → more rapid progression

2.131.) HYALINE MEMBRANE DISEASE

Prevalence	1-2% of newborns
Risk factors	o prematurity o diabetic mother
Prevention	• prenatal betamethasone accelerates lung maturation
Management	1. exogenous surfactant 2. mechanical ventilation (careful: avoid lung injury)

2.132.) HYPEREMESIS GRAVIDARUM

Prevalence	nausea and vomiting in 60-80% of pregnancies
Risk factors	o nulliparity o twin gestation o trophoblastic disease
Management	1. small frequent meals 2. avoid dehydration and nutritional depletion
Prognosis	• increased risk of fetal anomalies and growth • retardation if >5% weight loss

2.133.) ESSENTIAL HYPERTENSION

Prevalence	20% of population (of these 60% are salt-sensitive)
Risk factors	o family history o obesity o alcohol o excess dietary sodium

1. If no other risk factors for coronary artery disease:
- loose weight, exercise
- reduce Na^+ intake, increase K^+ intake

↓

2. Pharmacotherapy
- diuretics (or β-blocker, or calcium channel blocker)

↓

3. Pharmacotherapy
- combine diuretic with any of the other class drugs

2.134.) HYPERTROPHIC CARDIOMYOPATHY
(idiopathic hypertrophic subaortic stenosis)

Risk factors	o family history in 50% of cases (often autosomal dominant)
3° Prevention	• avoid strenuous exercise • avoid rapid standing • avoid inotropic drugs • avoid diuretics

---

1. Establish degree of abnormality
- echocardiography → thickness of left ventricular wall
- treadmill exercise testing → ischemia? hypotension?
- consider ambulatory ECG → arrhythmias

↓

2. Pharmacotherapy
- β-blocker

↓

3. Surgery
- for patients with severe symptoms despite medication
- left ventricular myotomy: removal of part of the septum

*Hypertrophic cardiomyopathy is a common cause of
sudden death in otherwise healthy young people.*

2.135.) IMMUNIZATIONS FOR ADULTS

dT	• every 10 years
measles	• if born before 1957 : assume "natural" immunity • if born after 1957 : recommend 2 doses • protective if given within 72 h of exposure • pregnant or immune compromised : give IgG
Pneumovax (give once)	• elderly > 65 years • chronic ill persons: COPD, HIV, CHF, DM etc. • prior to splenectomy
influenza (every autumn)	• elderly > 65 years • chronic ill persons: COPD, HIV, CHF, DM etc. • contacts and health care personnel

 No live vaccines for HIV positive infants or adults except MMR !

2.136.) <u>IMMUNIZATIONS FOR INFANTS</u>

	birth	2m	4m	6m	15m	4-6y
hepatitis B	●	●		●		
haemophilus influenzae		●	●	●	●	
oral polio		●	●		●	●
DTP / DTaP		●	●	●	○	○
MMR					●	●

 If mother is positive for HBsAg, give immunoglobulins to newborn.

2.137.) IMPETIGO

Prevalence	preschool-age children (highly communicable!)
Risk factors	o tropical climate o insect bites o minor trauma
Prevention	• good hygiene
Management	1. topical antibiotic cream 2. oral erythromycin

2.138.) ERECTILE IMPOTENCE

1. distinguish psychological from organic causes
- nocturnal penile tumescence

2. Search for organic causes
- peripheral vascular disease
- diabetic neuropathy
- endocrine
  - testicular failure
  - hyperprolactinemia

3. Treatment options
- Viagra (cGMP phosphodiesterase inhibitor)
- testosterone
- vacuum device to induce erection
- penile prothesis only if all others failed

2.139.) INFECTIOUS ARTHRITIS

Risk factors	o *N. gonorrhea*: 70% of cases
	o *Staphylococcus, Streptococcus, Haemophilus…*
	o trauma
	o joint prosthesis
Prevention	• STD prophylaxis

2.140.) INFERTILITY
(failure to become pregnant after 1 year of unprotected intercourse)

Prevalence	10-15% of all couples	
Risk factors	male factors	- 40%
	pelvic factors	- 30%
	ovulation failure	- 20%
	cervical factor	- 5%
	other	- 5%
Prevention	• prevent STDs and pelvic inflammatory disease	
Management	1. induce ovulation with clomiphene	
	2. artificial insemination	
	3. consider in vitro fertilization for:	
	- tubal disease	
	- oligospermia	
	- sperm antibodies	

Success rate of in vitro fertilization about 15%.
(multiple gestation in 25% of successful cases)

2.141.) INFLUENZA

Incidence	global epidemics (pandemics) every 10-15 years
Risk factors	o crowded conditions, dormitories, prisons etc. o chronic heart/lung diseases predispose to complications
Prevention	incubation period 1-5 days highest transmission at peak of symptoms **annual polyvalent vaccine for persons at risk:** • age >65 years • residents of chronic care facilities regardless of age • chronic heart and lung diseases • immunosuppression • diabetes • health care providers
Management	1. neuraminidase inhibitors effective when given early 2. symptomatic: fluids, antipyretics
Complications	bacterial pneumonia

Influenza A: antigenic shift due to gene reassortment between animal and human viruses.

Influenza B: antigenic drift due to spontaneous mutations.

206

2.142.) INSOMNIA

Prevalence	30% of adult population
Risk factors	o chronic illnesses o multiple drug use o obesity
Management	**SLEEP HYGIENE** **1.** daily exercise **2.** avoid caffeine **3.** avoid late night snacks **DRUGS** **4.** if necessary, use short-acting hypnotics

 Alcohol shortens sleep latency but hinders sleep maintenance. (frequent awakening after sleep onset)

2.143.) INTESTINAL OBSTRUCTION

Risk factors	o previous abdominal surgery (75% of cases) o external hernias o inflammatory bowel disease
Management	• if peritoneal signs → emergency surgery

 Carcinoma is the most common cause of colonic obstruction.

2.144.) <u>INTUSSUSCEPTION</u>

Risk factors	o Henoch-Schönlein purpura o leukemia, lymphoma o cystic fibrosis o recent upper respiratory infection
Management	• surgical emergency: prevent bowel infarction!

2.145.) <u>IRRITABLE BOWEL SYNDROME</u>

Prevalence	10-20% of adult population 20-50% of adults with IBS seek medical attention
Risk factors	o "learned illness behavior"?
Management	**diarrhea-predominant** • loperamide **constipation-predominant** • high-fiber diet • laxative: milk of magnesia ➢ consider low-dose antidepressant
Prognosis	lifelong condition, tends to lessen with age

2.146.) ITP

(idiopathic thrombocytic purpura)

Immune-mediated destruction of platelets.

Risk factors	**acute ITP:** children, female = male **chronic ITP:** adults, female > male
Management	**1.** avoid platelet inhibitors (aspirin) **2.** glucocorticoids if platelets < 30,000 **3.** intravenous IgG **4.** if bleeding → platelet transfusion **5.** splenectomy if medical therapy fails

2.147.) JUVENILE RHEUMATOID ARTHRITIS

Risk factors	o HLA-B27, DR4, DR5, DR6
Management	**1.** exclude uveitis → may lead to blindness **2.** glucocorticoids **3.** inject joint if only one or two are involved **4.** oral if systemic onset disease (Still's disease) **5.** add methotrexate or sulfasalazine if steroids are not enough
Prognosis	up to 80% remission, variable mobility poorest prognosis if rheumatoid factor positive and multiple joints affected

 Most cases of JRA are rheumatoid factor negative.

2.148.) KAPOSI SARCOMA

co-infection with human herpesvirus 8

Prevalence	1981: in 80% of AIDS patients 1992: in <10% of AIDS patients
Risk factors	HIV infection + male homosexuality (endemic Kaposi sarcoma in Zaire and Uganda)
Management	• cryotherapy or electrocoagulation • treatment of Kaposi sarcoma does not prolong life in patients with HIV infection

 HIV-related Kaposi sarcoma: mostly in homosexual men.

2.149.) KELOIDS

Prevalence	more common in black and Hispanic population
Risk factors	o family history o dark skin pigmentation o adolescence
Management	1. compression dressings 2. local steroid injections
Prognosis	• lesions tend to diminish over 6-12 months, • leaving a flat and shiny scar

2.150.) KIDNEY STONES

Risk factors	o high protein diet o low fluid intake o sedentary lifestyle o urinary tract infection **hereditary:** cystinuria
Prevention	• increase fluid intake (urine output > 3L/day) • diet: reduce oxalate, calcium, purines and Vit. C
Management	if < 4mm → may pass spontaneously if < 20 mm → lithotripsy if > 20 mm → surgery

2.151.) LACTOSE INTOLERANCE

Prevalence	American Indians: 100% African Americans: 80% Asians: 80% Caucasians: < 10%
Management	1. avoid milk (yogurt and cheese may be o.k.) 2. dietary lactase supplement 3. pre-hydrolyzed milk (LactAid)

2.152.) LEAD POISONING

Prevalence	~10% of preschool children have elevated blood lead levels!
Risk factors	o pica o pre-1970 houses (leaded paint) o lead-soldered plumbing o industrial soil
Management	1. immediate chelation: - EDTA - dimercaprol (BAL) 2. identify and eliminate source 3. report to OSHA if occupational

2.153.) LEGIONNAIRES' DISEASE

Risk factors	o smoking o alcohol abuse o chronic cardiopulmonary disease o immunosuppression
Prevention	• avoid inhalation of aerosols (keep water heaters > 160° F)
Management	➢ erythromycin
Prognosis	more severe than other "atypical pneumonias"

2.154.) LEUKEMIA, ACUTE

Incidence	most common type of cancer in children 80% ALL, 20% AML
Risk factors	o chromosomal abnormalities example: Philadelphia chromosome (t9:22) in ALL o radiation exposure o chemotherapy
Prognosis	**ALL in children:** expect long term survival **AML:** 60-80% remission rate 20-40% long term survival

Treatment is complex and depends on type and subtype. Below are just examples of some "classic" regimens:

---

1. Induction (to achieve remission)
- ALL: vincristine + prednisone + L-asparaginase
- AML: cytarabine + daunorubicin
- colony-stimulating factors to improve neutrophil count
- check bone marrow after 14 days

↓

2. CNS prophylaxis (to prevent leukemic meningitis in ALL)
- intrathecal methotrexate

↓

3. Consolidation therapy (to eradicate residual blast cells)
- same regimen as for induction, or single-agent high dose or...

↓

4. Maintenance therapy (to prevent relapse)
- mercaptopurine + methotrexate

213

2.155.) LEUKEMIA, CHRONIC

Incidence	CLL is the most common form of leukemia overall
Risk factors	o chromosomal abnormalities
Prognosis	**CML:** often converts to AML within 2 years with poor prognosis **CLL:** indolent for many years

---

CML

- consider allogenic bone marrow transplant for young patients

- Hydroxyurea
- interferon-α

- blast phase: treat like AML

CLL

- consider allogenic bone marrow transplant for young patients

- usually indolent, early treatment does not improve survival
- chemotherapy if anemia or neutropenia or other signs of disease progression develop:
  chlorambucil plus/minus glucocorticoid

2.156.) <u>LISTERIOSIS</u>

Risk factors	o high risk for fetuses and neonates
	o contact with infected animals
	
	o **food:** soft cheese
	            pâté
	            ready-to-eat pork
	            undercooked chicken

Prevention	• avoid handling livestock during pregnancy • avoid raw milk • avoid soft cheeses
Management	➤ penicillin

Pregnancy-associated:	mild disease in mother high risk of fetal demise
Neonatal infection:	high risk of meningitis high mortality

2.157.) LIVER CIRRHOSIS

Risk factors	o alcohol o viral hepatitis B and C o genetic (α1-antitrypsin deficiency, Wilson's etc.)
Prevention	• limit alcohol • hepatitis B immunization • avoid needle sharing • practice safe sex
Prognosis	<u>liver transplant</u>: 1-year survival: >80% 5-year survival: 60%

---

1. Diet
- normal caloric, normal protein diet
- reduce salt intake
- alcohol abstinence
- correct vitamin deficiencies

↓

2. Ascites
- diagnostic paracentesis → transudate
- reduce salt intake to 1g/day
- diuretics
- daily paracentesis
  (replace albumin IV)

↓

3. Surgical options
- consider TIPS: transjugular portosystemic stent
- liver transplant

2.158.) LUNG CANCER

Risk factors	o smoking o asbestos exposure
Prevention	• discontinue smoking • large scale screening (chest X-ray) is not recommended
Prognosis	• 5-year mortality >85%

1. Small cell carcinoma
- radiation plus chemotherapy
- consider cranial radiation to prevent CNS metastasis

↓

2. All other lung cancers
- early stage → lobectomy
- late stage → radiation plus chemotherapy

↓

3. Follow-up
- Physical exam including chest X-ray every 3 months

2.159.) LYME DISEASE

most common vector-borne infection in US

Risk factors	o tick infested areas o summer months
Prevention	• protective clothing
Management	➢ doxycycline

 Antibiotic prophylaxis after tick bite in otherwise asymptomatic persons is NOT recommended.

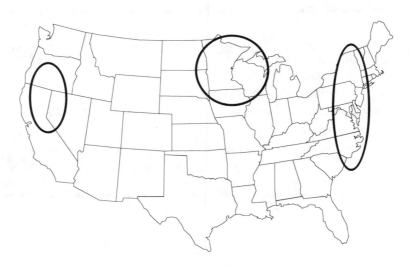

Disease is spreading and cases have been reported from most States.

2.160.) LYMPHOGRANULOMA VENEREUM

Risk factors	o unprotected intercourse o anal intercourse o tropical countries
Management	➢ doxycycline
Prognosis	• may result in scarring, strictures and fistulas if not treated adequately

2.161.) MAJOR DEPRESSIVE DISORDER

Prevalence	15-20% of population one episode during lifetime
Risk factors	o female o family history (25% chance of mood disorder if one parent has bipolar type I) (70% chance of mood disorder if both parents have bipolar type I)
Management	1. serotonin reuptake inhibitors are first choice (assess effectiveness after 4-6 weeks) 2. taper slowly 3. if patient had several episodes → give maintenance medication 4. if patient is psychotic → give separate antipsychotic 5. consider psychotherapy
Prognosis	- 50% chance of recovery during first year - better prognosis than bipolar disorder type I

2.162.) MALARIA

Risk factors	o transmitted by Anopheles mosquitos
Prophylaxis	• chloroquine for travel to Central America • mefloquine (or doxycycline) for all others
Management	*P. falciparum:* mefloquine *Others:* chloroquine **Prevention of relapse:** primaquine [1]

[1] eradicates liver schizont of *P. vivax* and *P. ovale*

 Mefloquine is effective in chloroquine resistant P. falciparum. It is safe during pregnancy.

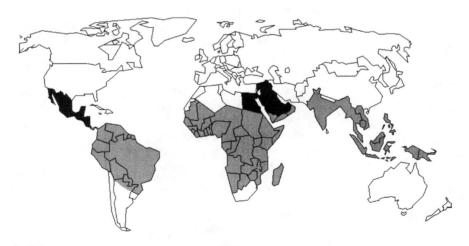

■ Chloroquine sensitive   ▨ Chloroquine resistant *P. falciparum*

220

2.163.) MARFAN'S SYNDROME

Risk factors	o family history (autosomal dominant)
Management	1. β-blockers may delay aortic dilatation 2. antibiotic prophylaxis for endocarditis if heart murmurs or valve abnormalities are present
Prognosis	- cardiovascular complications cause most of morbidity/mortality - normal life span with appropriate surgical interventions

2.164.) MASTALGIA

Prevalence	common in women with PMS
Risk factors	o methylxanthines: o coffee, tea, chocolate
Management	• usually remits spontaneously • for severe cases → consider tamoxifen
Prognosis	• premenstrual mastalgia increases with age and generally subsides with menopause

2.165.) <u>MELANOMA</u>

Risk factors	o fair complexion o history of blistering sunburn
Prevention	• sunscreens, hats… (most important during childhood and adolescence!)
Management	**1.** wide excision **2.** consider lymph node resection **3.** metastases: chemotherapy
Prognosis (AJCC)	<u>5-year survival</u> **Stage I and II** (localized) - 85% **Stage III** (one regional lymph node) - 50% (more than one regional lymph node) - 20% **Stage IV** (metastases) - <1%

2.166.) MÉNIÈRE'S DISEASE

Risk factors	o Caucasians o stress o allergy o increased salt intake
Management	**1.** reduce salt intake **2.** avoid ototoxic medications **3.** 5% of patients may require surgery for incapacitating vertigo
Prognosis	• vertigo tends to improve with time • hearing tends to decline with time

 Don't overlook acoustic tumors, which may produce a clinically identical picture.

2.167.) MENINGITIS

Risk factors	**bacterial:** immunosuppression
	                  head injury
	                  alcoholism

Management	**empirical therapy:** 3rd Generation cephalosporin + vancomycin (don't wait for results of CSF culture)
Prognosis	• bacterial more severe than viral!

223

2.168.) MENTAL RETARDATION

mild	(IQ < 70):
moderate	(IQ < 55):
severe	(IQ < 45):
profound	(IQ < 25):

Risk factors	~70% due to genetic abnormalities and congenital infections ~20% due to perinatal hypoxia, prematurity ~10% head trauma, CNS infections
Management	**mild:** basic job skills achievable **moderate:** group home living **severe:** need supervision **profound:** need extensive care

 A cause can be identified in 80% of severe cases and 50% of mild retardations.

2.169.) MIGRAINE

Risk factors	o family history, female > male o young age
Prophylactic	• daily propanolol if >2 attacks/month
Acute	➢ NSAIDs ➢ Ergot derivatives (not for patients with peripheral vascular disease) ➢ 5-HT agonists: sumatriptan

2.170.) <u>MITRAL STENOSIS</u>
common in patients with rheumatic heart disease

Risk factors	o history of rheumatic fever
Management	**1.** β-blockers to slow heart rate **2.** atrial fibrillation → anticoagulants (risk of thrombus) **3.** rheumatic fever → bacterial endocarditis prophylaxis **4.** consider balloon valvuloplasty in severe cases

2.171.) <u>MITRAL VALVE PROLAPSE</u>

Risk factors	o young females o cardiomyopathy
Management	**1.** β-blockers **2.** bacterial endocarditis prophylaxis if murmur present or valve appears thickened on echocardiogram

Endocarditis prophylaxis is NOT necessary if mid-systolic click is the only sign.

2.172.) INFECTIOUS MONONUCLEOSIS

Prevalence	90-95% of adult population seropositive
Risk factors	o higher socioeconomic groups [1] o college students o kissing
Management	➤ NSAIDs ➤ avoid aspirin (Reye syndrome)

[1] *higher probability of childhood infection in lower socioeconomic groups.*

2.173.) MGUS
(monoclonal gammopathy of unknown significance)

Prevalence	1% at age 60 years 3% at age 70 years
Management	annual quantitative measurement of M-protein
Prognosis	30% risk of multiple myeloma within 20 years

2.174.) <u>MULTIPLE MYELOMA</u>

Risk factors	o age o African Americans o family history
Management	1. if no symptoms ("smoldering"): observe 2. chemotherapy (melphalan + glucocorticoid) 3. young patients: consider high-dose chemotherapy with autologous stem cell transplantation

2.175.) <u>MULTIPLE SCLEROSIS</u>

Risk factors	o Northern European descent o living in temperate zone o family history
Management	• avoid stress from hot weather 1. glucocorticoids for acute attack 2. interferon-β to improve course of disease 3. baclofen to reduce muscle spasm 4. anticholinergics to reduce voiding reflex
Prognosis	**better if:** early onset relapsing-remitting course **worse if:** action tremors present primary progressive course

2.176.) <u>MUMPS</u>

Risk factors	o lack of immunization
Prevention	• MMR vaccine at 15 months and 4-6 years • virus is spread 2 days before to 10 days after parotitis
Management	• symptomatic
Prognosis	• encephalitis in 1% of cases • orchitis in 30% of postpubertal males (may decrease fertility, but sterility is rare)

 MMR vaccine NOT recommended for pregnant women, patients receiving glucocorticoids or immunosuppressed (except HIV).

2.177.) <u>MUSCULAR DYSTROPHY</u>

Duchenne is the most common form

Risk factors	Duchenne, Becker: x-linked recessive myotonic dystrophy: autosomal dominant
Prevention	Duchenne, Becker: determine maternal carrier status
Management	1. encourage exercise 2. avoid obesity 3. prednisone if there is a rapid decline in muscle strength

2.178.) <u>MYASTHENIA GRAVIS</u>

Risk factors	o other autoimmune diseases
Management	1. acetylcholinesterase inhibitors: pyridostigmine 2. glucocorticoids 3. thymectomy

*Thymus abnormalities (thymitis and thymoma) in 85% of patients.
Since most improve with thymectomy, this procedure should be
offered to all patients with myasthenia gravis.*

2.179.) NARCOLEPSY

Risk factors	o family history o head trauma o CNS infections
Management	1. avoid any long-distance driving 2. methylphenidate or other amphetamine-like stimulant

2.180.) NEURAL TUBE DEFECT

Risk factors	o 1st trimester valproic acid o folate deficiency o family history of spina bifida
Prevention	• folate supplementation during pregnancy
Management	• involve neurosurgeon, urologist and orthopedic
Prognosis	• >80% open neural tube infants will have normal IQ

2.181.) <u>NEUROBLASTOMA</u>

most common extracranial solid tumor of childhood

Risk factors	o genetic abnormalities o maternal phenytoin treatment o fetal alcohol syndrome
Management	**1.** surgical excision **2.** plus chemotherapy if advanced stage
Prognosis	survival 75% if age <1 year <25% if age >1 year

2.182.) <u>OBESITY</u>

Risk factors	o parental obesity o pregnancy o low socioeconomic status
Management	**1.** life-style modification **2.** exercise, low fat diet **3.** surgery only for select, severely obese patients
Prognosis	long term maintenance of weight loss extremely difficult

<u>Body Mass Index</u>: weight (kg) / height^2 (m^2)
overweight: BMI >25 kg/m^2
obese: BMI >30 kg/m^2

2.183.) ONYCHOMYCOSIS

Risk factors	o warmth o moisture o occlusive footwear
Prevention	• wear cotton socks • avoid wool or synthetic fibers
Management	1. topical or systemic antifungal (ketoconazole) 2. nail can be removed surgically or dissolved with urea
Prognosis	over 50% relapse

2.184.) OSGOOD SCHLATTER DISEASE

Risk factors	o male o rapid skeletal growth o repetitive jumping sports
Management	• avoid sports that stress quadriceps muscle (basketball, bicycle riding)
Prognosis	resolves after skeletal maturation

2.185.) OSTEOARTHRITIS

Risk factors	o age o obesity o trauma o (athletic activity ?)
Management	**1.** selective COX-2 inhibitor: rofecoxib **2.** intraarticular injection of glucocorticoid to reduce acute inflammation **3.** exercise to strengthen muscles and maintain mobility

2.186.) OSTEOMYELITIS

Risk factors	o sickle cell disease o IV drug use o open fractures
Management	**1.** Antibiotic therapy **acute osteomyelitis** • empirical antibiotic therapy against *Staph. aureus* (don't wait for results of culture) **chronic osteomyelitis** • identification of organism is important **2.** consider surgery to remove pus and necrotic tissue **3.** avoid weight bearing until healing

 MRI more sensitive than CT for diagnosis of osteomyelitis.

2.187.) OSTEOPOROSIS

Prevalence	up to 40% of elderly women
	up to 10% of elderly men
Risk factors	o menopause
	o inadequate dietary calcium/vit. D
	o excessive dietary phosphate
	o sedentary lifestyle
	o glucocorticoids
Management	1. hormone replacement therapy
	2. dietary calcium: 1g/day
	3. dietary Vit. D: 800 IU/day

Post-menopausal loss superimposed on age-related loss in females.

2.188.) OTITIS MEDIA

Risk factors	o day care setting
	o exposure to cigarette smoke
	o cleft palate
Prevention	• breast feeding
	• eliminate smoking in household
Management	• often resolves spontaneously
	• amoxicillin

Otitis media is often painless and should be suspected in children who "don't pay attention".

2.189.) OVARIAN CANCER

Risk factors	o low parity o late pregnancies o family history o Turner's syndrome
Prevention	• pregnancy or oral contraceptives reduce risk (by 30-60%)
Management	**1.** staging **2.** hysterectomy + bilateral salpingo-oophorectomy **3.** chemotherapy: cisplatin + cyclophosphamide

 Overall high mortality (60%) due to late detection.

2.190.) PANCREAS CANCER

Risk factors	o smoking o diabetes mellitus o chronic pancreatitis o African Americans
Management	**1.** if limited to head: pancreatomy or pancreaticoduodenectomy **2.** plus chemotherapy and/or radiation **3.** if inoperable: place stent to relief jaundice **4.** opioids for pain!

 70% occur in the pancreas head.

2.191.) PANCREATITIS

Risk factors	o alcoholism o cholelithiasis o ERCP
Prevention	• avoid alcohol
Management	**ACUTE** **1.** NPO **2.** admit patient to ICU **3.** vigorous IV fluid **4.** parenteral nutrition **5.** prophylactic antibiotics **6.** postpone cholecystectomy if possible **CHRONIC** **1. exocrine** insufficiency: oral enzymes **2. endocrine** insufficiency: may be deficient in both, insulin and glucagon **3.** advocate alcohol abstinence

RANSON'S CRITERIA (=poor prognosis):

at admission:
age > 55 years
WBC > 16,000/μL
glucose > 200 mg/dL
LDH > 400 IU/L
AST > 250 IU/L

within 48hours:
calcium < 8 mg/dL
hematocrit decreases > 10%
BUN increases > 5 mg/dL
albumin < 3.2 g/dL
pO_2 < 60 mmHg
fluid deficit > 4L

2.192.) <u>PATENT DUCTUS ARTERIOSUS</u>

Risk factors	o prematurity o high altitude o maternal rubella
Management	**1.** spontaneous closure after 3 months is rare **2.** should be surgically closed before age of 3 years

 Physiological closure should occur within 10-15h after birth.

Surgical closure recommended to prevent pulmonary hypertension and infectious endocarditis.

2.193.) <u>PELVIC INFLAMMATORY DISEASE</u>

Risk factors	o multiple sex partners o use of IUD o *C. trachomatis* and *N. gonorrhea* infection
Prevention	• practice safe sex • IUDs contraindicated if high risk sexual lifestyle
Management	**1.** get cervical culture **2.** antibiotics
Prognosis	• chronic pain in 20% • infertility in 15% • 6fold higher risk of ectopic pregnancy

2.194.) <u>PEPTIC ULCER DISEASE</u>

Prevalence	duodenal ulcer (DU) is clinically more common than gastric ulcer (GU) which often remains asymptomatic
Risk factors	o cigarette smoking o NSAIDs o glucocorticoids 100% of patients with DU harbor *H. pylori* 80% of patients with GU harbor *H. pylori* **no increased risk with:** o spicy food o alcohol, caffeine
Management	• gastric ulcers should be biopsied to exclude gastric cancer • *<u>H. pylori</u>* <u>eradication</u>: metronidazole + tetracycline + bismuth

 Most persons (60% > 60 years) harbor H. pylori but only some develop peptic ulcer disease.

238

2.195.) PERNICIOUS ANEMIA

Risk factors	o alcoholism
	o lack of vit. B12 (strict vegetarian diet)
	o gastrectomy
	o fish tapeworm *D. latum*
	o HLA-DR2 and HLA-DR4
Management	• lifelong parenteral Vit. B12
Prognosis	early detection of anemia can prevent later neurological complications
	anemia reversible with parenteral vit. B12
	neurological effects not reversible with vit. B12

2.196.) PERTUSSIS

Risk factors	o lack of immunization
Prevention	• DPT vaccine at 2,4,6 and 15 months and 6 years
Management	➤ erythromycin
Prognosis	very serious in infants <6 months

Prior to mass immunization, pertussis killed more children than measles, diphtheria, poliomyelitis and scarlet fever combined.

2.197.) PHENYLKETONURIA

Risk factors	o blond hair o blue eyes o fair skin
Management	**1.** routine neonatal screening (Guthrie test) **2.** low-phenylalanine diet at least until age 12 years
Prognosis	• may lose up to 50 IQ points during first year of life if undiagnosed

2.198.) PHEOCHROMOCYTOMA
most are benign

Prevalence	0.1% of hypertensive patients
Risk factors	o MEN 2 o neurofibromatosis
Management	**1.** <u>prior to surgery</u>: α-blocker: phenoxybenzamine β-blocker: propanolol **2.** surgical resection

2.199.) PLACENTA PREVIA

Risk factors	o prior placenta previa o previous cesarean section o previous induced abortions o multiple gestation
Management	**1.** hospitalize if possible **2.** have cross-matched blood ready **3.** Cesarean delivery for all cases

Perinatal mortality (15-20%) mainly due to prematurity.

2.200.) PLAGUE

Risk factors	o rats, fleas
	o Western States of US
Prevention	• avoid contact with vectors
	• vaccine is available for high risk people
Management	➤ streptomycin or gentamicin
Prognosis	15% fatality in US

 All cases need to be reported to the CDC.

2.201.) PNEUMONIA - BACTERIAL

Risk factors	o viral infections
	o hospitalization
	o elderly
	o alcohol/smoking
	o COPD
Prevention	• polyvalent pneumococcal vaccine
	• annual influenza vaccine for high risk persons
Management	**Empirical antibiotics:**
	• community acquired: clarithromycin or doxycycline
	• hospital acquired: broad spectrum cephalosporin or carbapenem.
	switch to selective antibiotic once pathogen has been identified

242

2.202.) <u>PNEUMONIA - MYCOPLASMA</u>

Risk factors	o army recruits o college students o other close communities
Management	➤ erythromycin

2.203.) <u>PNEUMONIA - PCP</u>

Prevalence	- most people have been exposed to PCP by age 3-4 years - 50% of AIDS patients experience PCP pneumonia
Risk factors	o immunodeficiency
Prevention	• CD4<200/µL: trimethoprim/sulfamethoxazole
Management	➤ trimethoprim/sulfamethoxazole ➤ pentamidine if above is not tolerated

First episode mortality was as high as 50% and is decreasing due to improved awareness and therapy.

2.204.) <u>PNEUMONIA - VIRAL</u>

90% of childhood pneumonias are viral

Risk factors	o immunocompromised o close quarters
Prevention	• hand washing
Management	• mostly symptomatic • avoid aspirin (Reye syndrome)

2.205.) <u>POLIOMYELITIS</u>

Incidence	5-10 cases/year in US (all due to live polio vaccine!)
Prevention	• consider inactivated polio vaccine (Salk)
Management	**1.** bed rest **2.** physical therapy **3.** intubation / tracheostomy may be needed
Complications	**meningitis** in1% of cases **paralysis** in <1% of cases

Many cases occur in contacts of persons who received the life oral polio vaccine (Sabin).

2.206.) <u>POLYCYSTIC KIDNEY DISEASE</u>

Prevalence	**adult form:** autosomal dominant **childhood form:** autosomal recessive
Associated with	**adult form:** intracranial aneurysms **childhood form:** hepatic fibrosis
Management	**1.** manage UTI and secondary renal hypertension **2.** dialysis **3.** kidney transplantation
Prognosis	**adult form:** 50% endstage renal disease at age 50y. **childhood form:** renal failure at <20 years of age

2.207.) <u>POLYCYSTIC OVARY DISEASE</u>
(Stein-Leventhal Syndrome)

Prevalence	common cause of oligomenorrhea/amenorrhea!
Risk factors	o obesity o hypertension o diabetes mellitus
Management	prevent endometrial and breast carcinoma (by reducing estrogen levels): ➢ oral contraceptives ➢ progesterone

245

2.208.) <u>POLYCYTHEMIA VERA</u>
most common myeloproliferative disorder

Risk factors	o Ashkenazi Jews o elderly
Management	• phlebotomy to reduce hematocrit to <45%
Complications	acute leukemia in up to 2% of patients

2.209.) <u>POLYMYOSITIS/DERMATOMYOSITIS</u>

Risk factors	o female o family history o other autoimmune diseases
Management	1. physical therapy 2. glucocorticoids (taper carefully after patient improves) 3. if unresponsive → methotrexate
Prognosis	50% full recovery 30% residual weakness 20% persistent active disease

2.210.) PORPHYRIA

enzymatic defect of heme biosynthesis

Risk factors	**genetic, attacks often triggered by:** ○ alcoholism ○ oral contraceptives ○ barbiturates ○ carbamazepine ○ sulfa drugs ○ (many more)
Management	1. avoid precipitating drugs 2. avoid sunlight if photosensitive 3. acute attack: IV heme analogue
Prognosis	• acute intermittent porphyria up to 25% mortality • other forms have excellent prognosis

2.211.) POST-TRAUMATIC STRESS DISORDER

Risk factors	○ childhood neglect/abuse may predispose
Prevention	• crisis intervention immediately after trauma reduces incidence of later post-traumatic stress syndrome
Prognosis	• delayed onset → worse prognosis • early treatment of acute phase → better prognosis

247

2.212.) PROSTATE CANCER

Prevalence	most common malignancy in men
	2nd most common cause of cancer death in men
Risk factors	o hormonal
	o carcinogenic toxins
	o African Americans
Prevention	• annual digital rectal exam for men >50
	• consider PSA screening

 PSA elevated in 65% of cases.
PSA also elevated in BPH and prostatitis.

---

1. Stage 1 (non-palpable)
2. Stage 2 (palpable)
- if patient's life expectancy is <10 years and if the tumor is of low-grade, consider observation only
- radical prostatectomy
- radiation
  (significant risk of impotence after radiotherapy)

---

3. Stage 3 (extends through capsule)
4. Stage 4 (metastasis)
- reduce androgens
  - bilateral orchiectomy
  - LHRH agonist
- chemotherapy

2.213.) PSEUDOMEMBRANOUS COLITIS

Risk factors	o antibiotics o bowel surgery o intestinal ischemia (shock etc.)
Prevention	• keep courses of antibiotics as brief as possible
Management	**1.** discontinue offending antibiotic **2.** if symptoms persist: metronidazole or vancomycin
Prognosis	- often resolves spontaneously once wide-spectrum antibiotic is discontinued - toxic megacolon has up to 30% mortality

The usual suspects: clindamycin, ampicillin and cephalosporins.

2.214.) PSITTACOSIS
Chlamydia psittaci infection

Risk factors	o poultry plants, pet shop owners (pet pigeon or parrot, chicken, turkey….)
Management	➤ prophylactic doxycycline if known exposure

All birds are susceptible and may or may not be sick.

249

2.215.) PSORIASIS

Risk factors	o family history **triggered by:** o local trauma/irritation o cold, stress o glucocorticoid withdrawal
2° Prevention	• avoid trigger factors • avoid antimalarial drugs
Management	➢ topical fluorinated glucocorticoids ➢ UVB phototherapy ➢ tar

2.216.) PUERPERAL INFECTION

Risk factors	o premature rupture of membranes o prolonged labor o Cesarean section o urinary tract infections
Prevention	• good prenatal care • patient education regarding rupture of membranes • antibiotic prophylaxis for C. section if at high risk
Management	➤ broad spectrum antibiotics if fever does not subside, consider: - retained products of conception - abscess - septic pelvic thrombophlebitis

2.217.) PULMONIC VALVE STENOSIS

Risk factors	o family history o other congenital heart defects
Management	• balloon valvuloplasty

2.218.) <u>PYELONEPHRITIS</u>

Prevalence	80% of cases are hospital acquired
Risk factors	o indwelling catheter o nephrolithiasis o diabetes mellitus
Prevention	• encourage fluid intake

Management	<u>empirical antibiotics against Enterobacteriaceae</u>
	• mild disease:
	   - oral fluoroquinolones
	• severe disease:
	   - 3rd generation cephalosporins
	   - gentamicin
	   - piperacillin

 10-15% of patients with indwelling catheters develop bacteriuria.

2.219.) PYLORIC STENOSIS

Risk factors	o Caucasians o first born o male
Management	• myotomy is effective in >99%

2.220.) RABIES

Risk factors	US: bats, skunks, raccoons outside of US: dogs
Management	post-exposure: 1. local wound cleansing 2. passive immunization on day 1 3. active immunization on days 1, 3, 7, 14 and 28

 Confine animal for 10 days. If it remains healthy, rabies is very unlikely.

2.221.) RAYNAUD'S PHENOMENON

Risk factors	o female o smoking o autoimmune connective tissue diseases
Management	**1.** avoid trauma to fingertips **2.** avoid exposure to cold **3.** stop smoking

 Raynaud's phenomenon is often the presenting symptom in scleroderma.

2.222.) REITER'S SYNDROME

Risk factors	o HLA-B27 o non-gonococcal urethritis o bacterial dysenteriae
Management	**1.** treat *Chlamydia* infection with tetracycline **2.** NSAIDs for arthritis **3.** physical therapy

2.223.) RENAL CELL CARCINOMA

Risk factors	o cadmium o asbestos o smoking o obesity
Management	• radical nephrectomy (kidney, adrenal gland, lymph nodes) • chemotherapy not very effective
Prognosis	<u>5-year survival</u> **Stage I** (confined to kidney) - 70% **Stage II** (extends through capsule) - 65% **Stage III** (involves hilar lymph nodes) - 20% **Stage IV** (invades adjacent organs) - 10%

2.224.) RETINA DETACHMENT

Risk factors	o myopia o trauma o retinal degeneration
Management	1. ophthalmic emergency 2. regular ophthalmologic exam if at high risk 3. seal retinal holes with laser

2.225.) RETROLENTAL FIBROPLASIA
leading cause of childhood blindness in US

Risk factors	o low birth weight o prematurity o supplemental oxygen
Prevention	• reduce risk factors a/w low birth weight: smoking, alcohol, drug abuse… • be careful with oxygen therapy • vitamin E (anti-oxidant)
Management	• may need laser coagulation to prevent retina detachment

2.226.) <u>REYE'S SYNDROME</u>
fatty liver plus encephalopathy

Risk factors	o Influenza B outbreaks o other viral infections o **aspirin, salicylates**
Management	**1.** glucose IV **2.** mannitol to reduce cerebral edema

2.227.) <u>RHEUMATOID ARTHRITIS</u>

Risk factors	o female o Native Americans o HLA-DR4
Management	**anti-inflammatory** ➤ NSAIDs ➤ glucocorticoids **disease-modifying drugs** ➤ methotrexate (low-dose) ➤ hydroxychloroquine ➤ sulfasalazine ➤ gold

 Disease-modifying drugs should be given early to slow the irreversible joint destruction!

2.228.) ROSEOLA
(exanthema subitum)

Prevalence	75% of children are seropositive for HHV-6 by age 1y.
Complications	encephalitis (rare)

2.229.) RUBELLA
(German measles)

Incidence	10-30% of young adults are susceptible in US !
Risk factors	o inadequate immunization
Prevention	• MMR vaccine at 15 months and 4-6 years (persons who receive vaccine do not transmit virus)
Complications	severe congenital disease (heart defects, cataract, glaucoma) occurs if maternal infection during first 2 months of pregnancy

> **Pregnant women exposed during first trimester:**
> 1. if seropositive: immunity is present - little risk
> 2. if seronegative: get second specimen in 4-6 weeks
>   if it converts: consider therapeutic abortion

2.230.) RUBEOLA

(measles)

Risk factors	o inadequate immunization
Prevention	• MMR vaccine at 15 months and 4-6 years
Management	• fluids • antipyretics
Complications	**encephalitis:** 1:1,000, 10% mortality **subacute sclerosing panencephalitis:** extremely rare

2.231.) SARCOIDOSIS

Risk factors	o African Americans (10 fold higher risk than Caucasians)
Management	• if extrapulmonary involvement → glucocorticoids
Prognosis	- spontaneous resolution in 80% - 20% active/recurrent disease

2.232.) <u>SCARLET FEVER</u>

Prevention	<ul><li>prophylactic penicillin after exposure is NOT recommended</li><li>treat group-A β-hemolytic streptococcal pharyngitis (mostly to prevent complications other than scarlet fever)</li></ul>
Management	<ul><li>➤ penicillin</li><li>children should not return to school until after 24h of treatment</li></ul>

2.233.) <u>SCHIZOPHRENIA</u>

Prevalence	1% of population at some point of their life
Risk factors	<ul><li>monozygotic twin concordance - 40%</li><li>dizygotic twin concordance - 10%</li><li>○ low socioeconomic status</li><li>○ severe stress often serves as a trigger</li></ul>
Management	**1.** **Neuroleptics (act on D-2 receptors)** Chlorpromazine: low-potency antipsychotic Haloperidol: high-potency antipsychotic Clozapine: fewer extrapyramidal side effects risk of agranulocytosis: monitor WBC **2.** **Maintenance** - for 1-2 years after first episode - IM depot haloperidol or fluphenazine **3.** Enroll patient in community-based support program

 Dyskinesias: *Acute dystonia (within hours of treatment) and Parkinsonism (weeks to months of treatment) are usually reversible. Tardive dyskinesia (after many months) is irreversible.*

2.234.) SEBORRHOIC DERMATITIS

Risk factors	o genetic predisposition o emotional stress triggers flare-ups
Management	1. selenium sulfide shampoos 2. ketoconazole cream 3. hydrocortisone cream
Prognosis	**infants:** resolves after 6-8 months **adults:** chronic

2.235.) SEPSIS

Risk factors	o age o indwelling catheters
Prevention	• pneumococcal vaccine for elderly • hand washing by hospital personnel • catheter care
Management	1. stabilize: airways, breathing, circulation 2. get blood cultures before antibiotics (aerobic and anaerobic cultures) 3. empiric antibiotics against: - *Staph. aureus* - *E.coli* - *Pseudomonas aeruginosa*

2.236.) SIALOADENITIS

Risk factors	o dehydration
	o hypercalcemia
Management	**1.** hydration
	2. suck on candy
	3. antistaphylococcal antibiotics

2.237.) SICKLE CELL ANEMIA

Prevalence	1:500 African Americans
	8% of African Americans have trait (heterozygous carriers)
Risk factors	**vaso-occlusive crisis**
	o dehydration
	o hypoxia
	aplastic crisis
	o severe infections
	o folic acid deficiency
	hemolytic crisis
	o bacterial infections
	o exposure to oxidant drugs

1. Prevent infections and complications
- penicillin prophylaxis for children
- pneumococcal vaccination
- bone pain plus fever → suspect osteomyelitis

- remove spleen if repeated infarction occurs

2. Anemic crisis
- bed rest, oxygen
- consider blood transfusion

2.238.) SILICOSIS

Risk factors	o metal mining o pottery making o sandstone cutting
Prevention	• avoid dust exposure • substitutes for silica
Complications	increased risk for tuberculosis

The classic "eggshell" pattern (calcification of hilar nodes) takes 10-20 years to develop.

2.239.) SLEEP APNEA

Prevalence	5% of population
Risk factors	o obesity o nasal obstruction o macroglossia
Management	• weight loss • avoid alcohol and sedatives • CPAP: continuous positive airway pressure at night • for severe cases: remove tonsils, adenoid, uvula

Obstructive sleep apnea is much more common than central sleep apnea.

Suspect in every patient with history of snoring and excessive daytime sleepiness.

2.240.) SQUAMOUS CELL CARCINOMA

Risk factors	o sun exposure o fair skin
Prevention	• sunscreens, hat…
Management	• excision (Mohs' method)
Prognosis	1-2% metastatic potential - higher if on ear and lips - lower if arising within actinic keratosis

2.241.) STASIS DERMATITIS/ULCER

Risk factors	o deep vein thrombosis o previous pregnancy o trauma o obesity o atopy
Management	**1.** elevate ankle **2.** compression stockings to prevent edema **3.** topical lubricant **4.** stasis ulcer: zinc oxide paste

2.242.) STROKE

Incidence	90% of cases due to ischemia-infarction
	10% of cases due to hemorrhage
Risk factors	o age
	o hypertension
	o smoking
	o diabetes
	o antiphospholipid antibodies
Prevention	• stop smoking
	• control blood pressure and diabetes
	• exercise

1. Acute stroke
- get CT to exclude intracranial hemorrhage
- consider tissue plasminogen activator
  (only for severe strokes in earliest phase)
- aspirin improves outcome

↓

2. Supportive care
- normalize blood pressure
- provide adequate nutrition
- watch for dehydration
- prevent deep vein thrombosis (heparin)

 Heparin and warfarin increase risk of intracranial hemorrhage.

2.243.) <u>SUBARACHNOID HEMORRHAGE</u>

Risk factors	o saccular aneurysm o polycystic kidney disease (adult type) o AV malformation o hypertension
Prevention	• prophylactic surgery of incidental aneurysms
Management	**1.** bed rest **2.** lower blood pressure **3.** phenytoin to prevent seizures **4.** aneurysms tend to rebleed → early surgery

Up to 3% of the population harbors saccular aneurysms.
(based on autopsy studies)

2.244.) <u>SUBDURAL/EPIDURAL HEMORRHAGE</u>

Risk factors	o motor vehicle accidents o falls o alcoholism o epilepsy
Prevention	• trauma prevention • avoid alcohol
Management	**1.** if minor: glucocorticoids, observe **2.** otherwise surgical evacuation

Subdural hemorrhage can occur without direct trauma.
(for example whiplash injuries)

2.245.) <u>SUDDEN INFANT DEATH SYNDROME</u>

Risk factors	o Minority groups o low socioeconomic status o **prone sleeping position**
Prevention	• healthy infants should be positioned on their side or back!
Management	• parents suffer from grief and feelings of guilt: provide supportive psychological counseling
Prognosis	siblings have a 2-3fold higher risk

A cause of death can be identified by autopsy in only 20% of cases.

2.246.) <u>SUICIDE</u>

Prevalence	- 2nd leading cause of death in adolescents - highest incidence in elderly >65 years - 80% of victims have seen physician in past 6 months
Risk factors	o depression o psychotic disorders o alcoholism o drug abuse o previous attempts
Management	**1.** hospitalize **2.** if overdose: remove drugs, prevent absorption, antidotes **3.** get psychiatric evaluation
Prognosis	10% of all attempts are "successful"

 Homicide is the leading cause of death in black male adolescents.

SOME ANTIDOTES:

INTOXICATION	ANTIDOTE
acetaminophen	N-acetylcysteine
opiates	naloxone
benzodiazepines	flumazenil
methanol, ethylene glycol	ethanol
CO	100% O_2
cyanide	amyl nitrate

2.247.) <u>SYPHILIS</u>

Risk factors	o multiple sexual partners o IV drug abuse o male homosexuality
Prevention	• safe sex practices
Management	➤ penicillin

Jarisch-Herxheimer reaction (fever, myalgia, headache) in 50% of patients within 2h of treatment.

2.248.) <u>SYSTEMIC LUPUS ERYTHEMATOSUS</u>

Risk factors	o African Americans o Asians, Hispanics o HLA-DR2, DR3, DQ3
Management	**SKIN** • avoid sun if photosensitive • malar rash: hydroxychloroquine **ARTHRITIS, SEROSITIS** • try NSAIDs first • short course of glucocorticoids **KIDNEYS** • renal biopsy to determine therapy and prognosis • high dose glucocorticoids

Drugs known to induce SLE are NOT contraindicated in patients with idiopathic SLE.

2.249.) <u>TEMPORAL ARTERITIS</u>

Risk factors	o age o polymyalgia rheumatica
Management	• high-dose glucocorticoid for 1 month • taper carefully when ESR declines
Prognosis	• high risk of blindness and stroke if untreated

2.250.) <u>TEMPOROMANDIBULAR JOINT SYNDROME</u>

Risk factors	o chronic teeth grinding o dental malocclusion o stress
Management	1. tension relief 2. orthodontics

2.251.) <u>TESTICULAR CANCER</u>

Risk factors	o age 20-40 years o Caucasians o history of cryptorchidism o higher socioeconomic status o unmarried
Management	**SEMINOMAS** • orchiectomy plus radiotherapy • chemotherapy for advanced stages **NON-SEMINOMAS** • orchiectomy plus chemotherapy
Prognosis	- infertility - 70-90% cure, even in advanced cases

 Consider cryopreservation (sperm-bank) before beginning treatment.

2.252.) <u>TESTICULAR TORSION</u>

Risk factors	o adolescence o winter season
Management	**1.** distinguish from inflammation (Doppler ultrasound) **2.** immediate surgery
Prognosis	• <85% testicular salvage if duration >6 hours • 2/3 of salvaged testicles will atrophy later

 Any child/adolescent with scrotal pain should be assumed to have torsion unless proven otherwise.

271

2.253.) <u>TETANUS</u>

Risk factors	o burns o frost bite o skin ulcers o drug addiction
Prevention	• maintain active immunization (toxoid every 10 years)
Management	1. give anti-tetanus immune-globulin immediately 2. IV glucocorticoids immediately 3. diazepam to reduce spasms

MANAGEMENT OF TETANUS-PRONE WOUNDS:

Immunization History	Tetanus Toxoid	Anti-Tetanus Immune Globulin
<u>3 prior doses</u>		
• clean minor wound	yes if > 10 years	no
• other wound	yes if > 5 years	no
<u>immunization unknown or less than 3 doses</u>		
• clean minor wound	yes	no
• other wound	yes	yes

2.254.) THALASSEMIA

Risk factors	o Mediterranean o Middle East o Southeast Asia
Management	**1.** prompt treatment of infections **2.** dental checkups **3.** reduce risk for bone fractures
Prognosis	**Thalassemia major:** life expectancy < 20 years **Thalassemia minor:** normal life expectancy

Hemoglobinopathies are extremely heterogeneous on the molecular level (over 600 known mutations).

2.255.) THROMBOPHLEBITIS

Risk factors	o immobilization o IV catheters (especially lower extremities) o IV drug abuse
Prevention	• replace IV cannulas every 48-72 hours
Management	• warm compresses • NSAIDs • antibiotics are not needed

2.256.) <u>THYROID CANCER</u>

Incidence	papillary > follicular > anaplastic
Risk factors	**papillary carcinoma:** head and neck irradiation **medullary carcinoma:** MEN 2

Management	**1.** thyroidectomy
	  - protect parathyroids
	  - watch out for recurrent laryngeal nerves!
	2. radioactive iodine to destroy thyroid remnants
	3. give thyroid hormone to suppress TSH
	4. for anaplastic cancer → add radiation therapy

Prognosis	papillary (best) > follicular > anaplastic

2.257.) <u>TOURETTE'S SYNDROME</u>
motor and vocal tics

Risk factors	o male o family history (up to 30% have motor ticks)
Management	• α-blockers (clonidine) to suppress tics
Prognosis	50% improve spontaneously during adolescence

 Intelligence does not deteriorate!

2.258.) TOXIC SHOCK SYNDROME

Risk factors	o young women o tampons o nasal packing
Prevention	• frequent tampon change
Management	**1.** penicillin or clindamycin **2.** IV immune globulins **3.** surgical intervention for TSS due to necrotizing fasciitis

>90% of female adults have anti-TSS-toxin antibodies.

2.259.) TOXOPLASMOSIS

Risk factors	<u>transplacental transmission</u>: **1ˢᵗ trimester:** lowest transmission rate (15%) severe neonatal disease **3ʳᵈ trimester:** highest transmission rate (65%) asymptomatic neonates
Prevention	• avoid cat feces • avoid raw meat, raw eggs
Management	➢ pyrimethamine plus sulfadiazine
Prognosis	- acute toxoplasmosis is usually asymptomatic - high risk of encephalitis in AIDS patients

Women who are seropositive before pregnancy are protected against acute infection (i.e. no risk of congenital disease for fetus).

2.260.) TRICHINOSIS

Risk factors	o undercooked pork
	o undercooked wild game
Management	• self-limited disease
	➢ NSAIDs for muscle pain
Prognosis	• most infections asymptomatic
	• rarely enteritis or myositis

2.261.) TRICHOMONIASIS

Risk factors	o multiple sex partners
Prevention	• safe sex practice
	• treat partner
Management	➢ metronidazole

 Most men are asymptomatic.

2.262.) <u>TRISOMY 21</u>
(Down syndrome)

Risk factors	**maternal age:** 1:2000 at age 20 1:200 at age 35 1:20 at age 45
Prevention	**triple screen test** for all pregnant women - AFP, hCG, estriol **amniocentesis** at 13-15 weeks if high risk
Prognosis	• 1% recurrence risk (much higher if due to translocation) • premature aging • clinical Alzheimer's disease after age 35 in 30% of cases

 Risk of fetal loss with amniocentesis is 0.5%.

2.263.) <u>TUBERCULOSIS</u>

Most infected people never develop active tuberculosis. However, multi drug-resistance is increasingly common and TB remains a major health threat worldwide.

Risk factors	o urban, homeless
	o close contact with infected
	o immunosuppression
Prevention	• annual PPD skin test for high risk persons
	• BCG vaccine has inconsistent efficacy

---

1. Diagnosis
- Chest X-ray
- Get several sputums for culture and sensitivity testing
- Notify local health department

↓

2. Latent tuberculosis
- **Isoniazid prophylaxis if:**
  PPD > 15 mm in low risk persons
  PPD > 10 mm in high risk persons
  PPD >   5 mm in HIV patients

↓

3. Active tuberculosis
- **goal:** prevent treatment failure due to acquired drug resistance
- <u>**4-drug regimen:**</u>
- isoniazid + rifampin + pyrazinamide + ethambutol
- monthly follow-up sputum cultures
- patient compliance is most important!

Previous BCG vaccination produces skin reactivity, but induration >15 mm should be considered positive.

2.264.) <u>TULAREMIA</u>

Risk factors	outdoor work **reservoir:** white rabbits, small game… **vectors:** ticks, fleas…
Prevention	• tick repellents • avoid contact with ill game
Management	➢ streptomycin

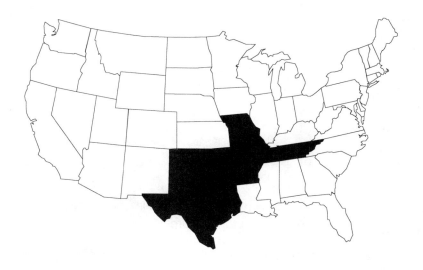

2.265.) TURNER'S SYNDROME

Prevention	• prenatal detection for couples with chromosome translocations
Management	**Genetic counseling:** • low fertility rate • if pregnant: high risk of chromosomal abnormalities in offspring

2.266.) TYPHOID FEVER
(S. typhi, S. paratyphi A and B, S. typhimurium)

Risk factors	o travel to tropical countries o contaminated water o human carriers
Prevention	• avoid tap water • avoid salads, raw vegetables • avoid unpeeled fruits • vaccine if traveling to high-risk endemic area
Management	➤ chloramphenicol ➤ if resistant: ciprofloxacin

 Non-typhoid salmonellosis is much more common in US than typhoid fever.

2.267.) TYPHUS FEVER

Risk factors		RESERVOIR	VECTOR
	epidemic typhus:	humans	lice
	scrub typhus:	rodents	mites
	endemic (murine) typhus:	rodents	fleas

Prevention	• sanitation • avoid vectors

Management	➤ all *Rickettsia* are sensitive to tetracycline

Prognosis	epidemic typhus:	50% mortality untreated
	scrub typhus:	30% mortality untreated
	endemic typhus:	<2% mortality untreated

2.268.) ULCERATIVE COLITIS

Risk factors	o Caucasians o Jews o family history o major psychological stress → trigger
Prognosis	75% will relapse 20% will require colectomy

---

1. Medical therapy
- sulfasalazine (5-ASA is the active moiety)
- if unresponsive: oral glucocorticoids
- acute and severe colitis: IV glucocorticoids

↓

2. Surgical therapy
Indications:
- colitis unresponsive to medical therapy
- toxic megacolon unresponsive to antibiotics

Colonoscopy should be performed every 1~2 years to detect dysplasia or colon cancer. If high-grade dysplasia, consider colectomy.

2.269.) URINARY INCONTINENCE

Risk factors	o age o multiparity o diabetes
Prevention	• Kegel exercises after birth of children
Management	1. "bladder training": pelvic muscle exercises 2. anticholinergic drugs 3. consider surgery

2.270.) URINARY TRACT INFECTION

Risk factors	o diabetes mellitus o pregnancy o prostate hypertrophy o sexual activity o catheter use
Prevention	• maintain good hydration • sparse use of catheters
Management	empirical antibiotics: ➢ trimethoprim-sulfamethoxazole • if signs of pyelonephritis: get urine culture before starting antibiotics

2.271.) <u>UTERINE MYOMAS</u>

Prevalence	40% of women >50 years, most are asymptomatic
Risk factors	o African Americans o (estrogen ?)
Management	**1.** if asymptomatic : no treatment necessary **2.** if mild symptoms: oral contraceptives or progesterone **3.** if severe symptoms: myomectomy or hysterectomy
Prognosis	• usually decrease in size after menopause • 10% recurrence following myomectomy

 Caution: may mask other (potentially lethal) pelvic tumors.

2.272.) <u>VAGINAL CARCINOMA</u>

Risk factors	**squamous carcinoma**
	   o HPV
	   o smoking
	
	clear cell carcinoma
	   o daughters of mothers who took DES [1]

Prevention	• annual Pap smear
Management	1. radiation 2. if localized to upper 1/3 : radical hysterectomy with upper vaginectomy
Prognosis	<u>5-year survival</u> **Stage I** (limited to mucosa) - 60% **Stage II** (invades subvaginal tissue) - 40% **Stage III** (extends to pelvic wall) - 20% **Stage IV** (invades rectum or bladder) - 3%

[1] *up to 0.1% of exposed female fetuses.*

2.273.) VENTRICULAR SEPTAL DEFECT
most common congenital heart defect

Risk factors	o increased risk if sibling affected
Prevention	• for adults: reduce risk factors for MI
Management	1. small defects may be left unrepaired. 2. surgical closure should be performed before pulmonary hypertension develops! 3. if pulmonary vascular disease develops, heart-lung transplant becomes the only option.
Prognosis	**congenital:** 50% will close spontaneously

2.274.) VITILIGO
loss of melanin pigment

Risk factors	o family history in 30% o often triggered by stressful event
Management	1. PUVA: psoralen plus UV light 2. topical glucocorticoids 3. avoid sun exposure while treated!

2.275.) WARTS

(verruca vulgaris)

Risk factors	o immunosuppression o atopic dermatitis o locker rooms
Prevention	• avoid wound fluid after cryotherapy
Management	**1.** cryotherapy **2.** keratolytics: salicylic acid plasters
Prognosis	warts often regress spontaneously

2.276.) WILMS' TUMOR

nephroblastoma

Risk factors	o aniridia o cryptorchidism o hypospadia o other urogenital abnormalities
Management	**1.** surgical resection **2.** adjuvant chemotherapy or radiation
Prognosis	**"favorable histology":** 90% survival **"unfavorable histology":** 50-70% survival

Second most common abdominal tumor in children.
(after neuroblastoma)

287

2.277.) ZOLLINGER-ELLISON SYNDROME

Risk factors	o MEN 1 (up to 50% of cases)
2° Prevention	• screen all first degree relatives for MEN
Management	**1.** get CT or scintigraphy if no metastases → attempt surgical cure **2.** proton pump inhibitors: omeprazole **3.** if gastrectomy is necessary: replace B12, iron...
Prognosis	surgical cure in 30% of cases 10-year survival 50%

Gastrinomas arise in the pancreas or duodenum and are slow growing.

2/3 are malignant → liver metastases

ABBREVIATIONS

a/w	associated with	IUD	intrauterine device
AA	amyloid A protein	IVP	intravenous pyelography
ACE	angiotensin converting enzyme	LBBB	left bundle branch block
AFP	alpha fetoprotein	LDL	low density lipoproteins
AIP	acute intermittent porphyria	LES	lower esophageal sphincter
AJCC	Am. Joint Commission on Cancer	LFT	liver function tests
AL	amyloid light chains: κ, λ	LMN	lower motor neuron
ANA	antinuclear antibodies	MALT	mucosa-associated lymphoid tissue
ANLL	acute non-lymphocytic leukemia	MCHC	mean corpuscular hemoglobin
ASD	atrial septal defect		concentration
ATN	acute tubular necrosis	MCV	mean corpuscular volume
BCG	bacillus Calmette-Guérin	MEN	multiple endocrine neoplasia
BP	blood pressure	MGUS	monoclonal gammopathy of
BPH	benign prostate hyperplasia		unknown significance
CDC	Center for Disease Control	MI	myocardial infarction
CHF	congestive heart failure	MR	mitral regurgitation
CMML	chronic myelomonocytic	MS	mitral stenosis
	leukemia	NIDDM	non-insulin-dependent diabetes
CMV	cytomegalovirus		mellitus
COPD	chronic obstructive pulmonary	OSHA	Occupational Safety and Health
	disease		Administration
COX	cyclooxygenase	PCP	Pneumocystis carinii pneumonia
CPK	creatine phosphokinase	PCT	porphyria cutanea tarda
CVA	cerebrovascular accident	PFT	pulmonary function tests
CXR	chest X-ray	PID	pelvic inflammatory disease
DES	diethylstilbestrol	PMS	premenstrual syndrome
DIC	disseminated intravascular	PPD	purified protein derivative
	coagulation	PSA	prostate specific antigen
DM	diabetes mellitus	RBBB	right bundle branch block
DPT	diphtheria-pertussis-tetanus	RSV	respiratory syncytial virus
DVT	deep vein thrombosis	SBFT	small bowel follow through
EBV	Epstein-Barr virus	STD	sexually transmitted disease
EEE	eastern equine encephalitis	TIA	transient ischemic attack
ENG	electronystagmography	TIBC	total iron binding capacity
ERCP	endoscopic retrograde	TTP	thrombotic thrombocytopenic
	cholangiopancreatography		purpura
ESR	erythrocyte sedimentation rate	UGI	upper gastrointestinal
FNA	fine needle aspiration	UTI	urinary tract infection
GN	glomerulonephritis	UMN	upper motor neuron
HDL	high density lipoproteins	VDRL	Venereal Disease Research
HPV	human papilloma virus		Laboratories
IDDM	insulin-dependent diabetes mellitus	VSD	ventricular septal defect
ITP	idiopathic thrombocytopenic	WPW	Wolff-Parkinson-White syndrome
	purpura		

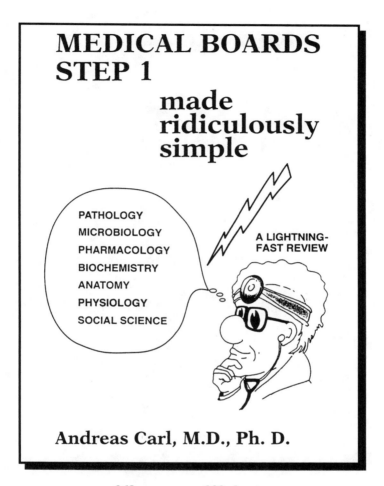

MEDICAL BOARDS STEP 1

made ridiculously simple

PATHOLOGY
MICROBIOLOGY
PHARMACOLOGY
BIOCHEMISTRY
ANATOMY
PHYSIOLOGY
SOCIAL SCIENCE

A LIGHTNING-FAST REVIEW

Andreas Carl, M.D., Ph. D.

368 pages - 333 charts

♦ Covers all Basic Medical Sciences in a Chart Format.

♦ Emphasizes Clinical Correlations

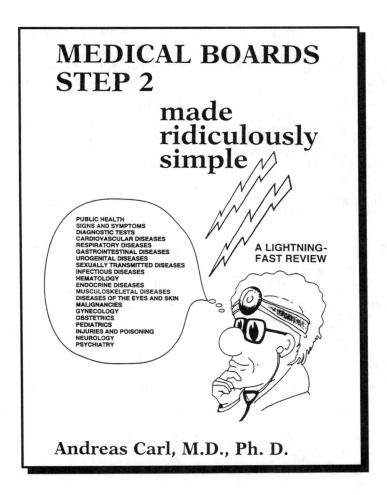

MEDICAL BOARDS STEP 2

made ridiculously simple

PUBLIC HEALTH
SIGNS AND SYMPTOMS
DIAGNOSTIC TESTS
CARDIOVASCULAR DISEASES
RESPIRATORY DISEASES
GASTROINTESTINAL DISEASES
UROGENITAL DISEASES
SEXUALLY TRANSMITTED DISEASES
INFECTIOUS DISEASES
HEMATOLOGY
ENDOCRINE DISEASES
MUSCULOSKELETAL DISEASES
DISEASES OF THE EYES AND SKIN
MALIGNANCIES
GYNECOLOGY
OBSTETRICS
PEDIATRICS
INJURIES AND POISONING
NEUROLOGY
PSYCHIATRY

A LIGHTNING-
FAST REVIEW

Andreas Carl, M.D., Ph. D.

381 pages - 275 charts

♦ Systematic Review of Diseases and Organ Systems in Chart Format

♦ Patient Management and Therapy.